ORGANIZE YOUR EMOTIONS, OPTIMIZE YOUR LIFE

Decode Your Emotional DNA—and Thrive

MARGARET MOORE, MBA, EDWARD PHILLIPS, MD, AND JOHN HANC

WILLIAM MORROW

An Imprint of HarperCollins*Publishers*

ORGANIZE YOUR EMOTIONS, OPTIMIZE YOUR LIFE. Copyright © 2016 by Harvard University. All rights reserved. Printed in the United States of America. No part of this book may be used or reproduced in any manner whatsoever without written permission except in the case of brief quotations embodied in critical articles and reviews. For information address HarperCollins Publishers, 195 Broadway, New York, NY 10007.

HarperCollins books may be purchased for educational, business, or sales promotional use. For information please e-mail the Special Markets Department at SPsales@harpercollins.com.

FIRST EDITION

Designed by Diahann Sturge

Library of Congress Cataloging-in-Publication Data has been applied for.

ISBN 978-0-06-241977-4

16 17 18 19 20   OV/RRD   10 9 8 7 6 5 4 3 2 1

CONTENTS

ORGANIZE YOUR EMOTIONS, OPTIMIZE YOUR LIFE

INTRODUCTION

Ask yourself this question: Just how stressed out are you?

A. Not at all. I'm cool, calm, and collected. I feel that I'm in tune with myself and my needs. I know where I'm going, and I'm on my way. No sweat!

B. I think I have a handle on everything, but there are days when my blood pressure soars, my mood is foul, and I'm ready to scream at the first person who cuts me off on the way to work!

C. I feel like I'm in a constant state of frenzy. I'm totally stressed out . . . at home, on the job, even on vacation! I'm anxious, I'm nervous, and I'm agitated. . . . Oh, did I say I'm stressed out? Help!

If you answered A, B, or C, this book is for you! We'll explain why in a minute, but first, here are a couple more questions—and a clarification.

Stress is a term that's thrown around a lot. Sometimes there are good reasons to be stressed. You could be stressed because you've just been through a divorce, you lost your job, or you suffered through some other personal or professional crisis. That's to be expected. Sometimes, though, the feeling of being stressed is a manifestation of deeper issues. Perhaps you feel that way because, like so many of us, you don't get the sense that your life is headed in the right direction or that you're living up to your capabilities.

Let's find out your current state of mind with our next question: How much of the time over the past thirty days have you felt this way?

1. Cheerful
2. In good spirits
3. Extremely happy
4. Calm and peaceful
5. Satisfied
6. Full of life

You can answer:

A. All the time
B. Some of the time
C. Hardly ever

How many As did you get? None? Did you get mostly Bs and Cs? You will *definitely* want to read on. Here's our last question (actually, there are two). This pair of questions zeroes in on the heart of the matter.

Do you feel like you're firing on all cylinders in your life? Do you feel as if you're engaged and challenged, but calm and generally satisfied?

A. Yes, my life is sailing along smoothly, thank you.
B. There's a lot of turbulence, but I'm still airborne.
C. I'm grounded. I think my cylinders are clogged.

Okay, that's the end of our questions (for now). If you had a lot of Bs and Cs in your answers, you're like the majority of Americans. You are, to use psychological terms, more likely to be surviving or languishing, not thriving.

This book can change all that. This book can help you reduce stress and tame the frenzy, yes. But more importantly, this book—and the groundbreaking theory behind it—can help you flourish, thrive, and *soar.*

And the way we point you skyward is by first looking inward.

THRIVING INSTEAD OF
LANGUISHING OR SURVIVING

How do we define *emotional well-being?* In his influential 2002 paper "The Mental Health Continuum: From Languishing to Flourishing in Life," social scientist Corey L. M. Keyes of Emory University examines various definitions of *mental health* and determines that individuals who seem to be functioning best have warm and trusting relationships, have a direction in life, are able to shape their environment to satisfy their needs, and have a degree of self-determination.

These individuals also appear to like most parts of themselves. (Yes, that's *parts,* plural. This is an important point, and we'll come back to it.) In addition, those who are flourishing feel that they are contributing to and are engaged with society, and they have the ability and the willingness to adapt to change.

"To be flourishing," Keyes writes, "is to be filled with positive emotions and to be functioning well, psychologically and socially." On the other hand, those who are languishing, Keyes posits, have feelings of "emptiness and stagnation, constituting a life of quiet despair." These individuals describe themselves and their lives as "hollow . . . empty . . . a shell . . . a void."

Since the dawning of the twenty-first century, Americans have lived through nearly fifteen years of war and a Great Recession, have endured a polarized political climate, and have witnessed exciting but disruptive technological changes. In this new century, many people's dreams and expectations have diminished; they have been downsized to the same extent as the American workforce. As we write this, it's probably safe to say that more people today would describe themselves as languishers than flourishers. Many polls have confirmed this perception, most notably the annual Gallup-Healthways Well-Being Index, which concluded in 2010 that in the wake of the recession "Americans' emotional recovery is on shaky ground." Increasing economic worries and health problems were cited as the primary culprits for this state of affairs, not surprisingly.

You might be one of those who feel that they are languishing. Or you might be somewhere in the middle: you might feel that you are simply surviving. You're getting by, you're making the best of things, but you're certainly not filled with positive emotions. And you're certainly not flourishing.

The goal of this book is to help you get to that place where you can *thrive*. When you thrive, you perform at the best possible level. And the more you thrive, the better your brain functions, and consequently, you're more creative, resourceful, and open-minded. When you thrive, you perform better at work and interact better at home. Your health improves. You enjoy life more. When you're thriving, your stress level is down, because your confidence and your sense of self-mastery are way up. When you're thriving, the frenzy is tamed by a poised, confident mind.

So how does one leave languishing and surviving in the dust

and get to this exalted state of flourishing? Does one win the lottery? Get a big promotion? Find Mr. or Ms. Right?

All of those might help, but they're external factors, often as far beyond your control as world peace, global warming, traffic jams, or stock market crashes—all of which can affect you in both the short and long term, as well.

Rather, getting to this exalted state, this flourishing, is better achieved by managing *yourself*—your emotions, your needs, and your drives and motivations. All the varied aspects of your own personality. This self-management is the key to reducing the stress and taming the frenzy.

When you think about it, this makes perfect sense. News flash: you can't control what your boss will say or do today or the sudden emergence of some new technology, one that you must master in order to do your job. You can't control the weather or interest rates or the events in Washington, D.C., or the Middle East. Heck, you can't even control everything that goes on under your own roof! (Parents of teenagers know just what we're talking about here.) These are all *external* factors.

What you *do* have control over is yourself. And as much as we would like to think that the answer to our challenges is more money, more time, more food, or more whatever, it's not out there. It's in *here* (at this point, please gently tap your noggin). That's where the answers to a happier, more productive, more positive, and less stressful life can be found.

This is true even if you're someone who feels like you're on top of your game. You can feel even better if you follow some of the recommendations in this book.

We will show you some examples of what that state of thriving looks like, that point where you feel like you're gliding through life, like you're out of the weeds (a source of confusion) and are soaring through clear blue skies and reaching your potential, engaging and utilizing your abilities to the max. The state of thriving is attained when you are flexible enough to handle any rough patches without ruffling your feathers.

Yes, that is achievable, and we can help you get there. We can help you spread your wings and thrive.

But first, let's check your altitude level to see where you are today, to see how satisfied you are with your life right now.

Are You Thriving, Just Surviving, or Languishing?

Review these ten statements to find out. Read each statement and then determine the degree to which it reflects your experience, using the scale following each statement. Keep a tally of the points earned for each response as you go.

I feel like I am free to decide for myself how to live my life.

___ Very often or always true (5 points)

___ Often true (4 points)

___ Sometimes true (3 points)

___ Rarely true (2 points)

___ Very rarely or never true (1 point)

I am satisfied with my life. (Since precision matters in this exercise, note that *Merriam-Webster's Collegiate Dictionary,* eleventh edition, defines *satisfaction* as "fulfillment of a want or need; the quality or state of being satisfied: contentment.")

___ Very often or always true (5 points)

___ Often true (4 points)

___ Sometimes true (3 points)

___ Rarely true (2 points)

___ Very rarely or never true (1 point)

I feel as though I have a clear sense of purpose.

    __ Very often or always true (5 points)

    __ Often true (4 points)

    __ Sometimes true (3 points)

    __ Rarely true (2 points)

    __ Very rarely or never true (1 point)

I derive a sense of accomplishment from what I do.

    __ Very often or always true (5 points)

    __ Often true (4 points)

    __ Sometimes true (3 points)

    __ Rarely true (2 points)

    __ Very rarely or never true (1 point)

I have good relationships, that is, relationships characterized by mutual caring, appreciation, collaboration, and respect.

    __ Very often or always true (5 points)

    __ Often true (4 points)

    __ Sometimes true (3 points)

    __ Rarely true (2 points)

    __ Very rarely or never true (1 point)

I perceive my feelings and emotions without being hijacked by them.

    __ Very often or always true (5 points)

    __ Often true (4 points)

    __ Sometimes true (3 points)

    __ Rarely true (2 points)

    __ Very rarely or never true (1 point)

I pay attention to how my emotions affect my thoughts and behavior.

___ Very often or always true (5 points)

___ Often true (4 points)

___ Sometimes true (3 points)

___ Rarely true (2 points)

___ Very rarely or never true (1 point)

When I feel negative emotions, I "step back" and am aware of the emotions without getting taken over by them.

___ Very often or always true (5 points)

___ Often true (4 points)

___ Sometimes true (3 points)

___ Rarely true (2 points)

___ Very rarely or never true (1 point)

I experience a good level of positive emotions (e.g., cheerfulness, contentedness, joyfulness, energy, optimism, excitement).

___ Very often or always true (5 points)

___ Often true (4 points)

___ Sometimes true (3 points)

___ Rarely true (2 points)

___ Very rarely or never true (1 point)

I know what makes me thrive. (Note that *Merriam-Webster's Collegiate Dictionary,* eleventh edition, defines *thrive* as "to grow vigorously: flourish.")

___ Strongly agree (5 points)

___ Moderately agree (4 points)

___ Slightly agree (3 points)

___ Moderately disagree (2 points)

___ Strongly disagree (1 point)

Add up your score! If you have a score of 40 or above, you are a Thriver. Congratulations. If your score is 39 or below, you are a Survivor or a Languisher (you know which).

Keep in mind that this isn't an official mental health assessment; it is simply a guide. Mostly, we want to get you thinking about how you are doing and what makes you thrive. No matter how you scored, this book has something to offer you. If you are a Survivor or a Languisher, you can unlock your potential and become a Thriver. And if you're a Thriver, you can soar even higher.

THE SURVIVAL MENTALITY

When you're down, when you're in survival mode, when you're blue, it's easy to feel like everyone else is not. You may think that you're one of the few who are in a state of frenzy and constantly stressed out, who feel like they are getting nowhere in life.

Not so. In his study "The Mental Health Continuum," Keyes estimates that only about 17 percent of Americans consider themselves truly thriving. At the other end of the spectrum, about 26 percent are languishing or depressed. And the majority of Americans, 57 percent, are surviving.

Sobering statistics. But as we said, there is a way to get yourself out of these doldrums. There is a way to lighten the stress and tame the frenzy. There is a way to thrive. Allow us to introduce the team that will help you navigate the journey from surviving to thriving.

Margaret Moore, aka Coach Meg, is cofounder of the Institute of Coaching at McLean Hospital, a Harvard Medical School affiliate. Moore has combined two careers—the first one as a biotechnology executive who launched a neuroscience-based biotech company and the second as a coach, leader, and trainer. As the founder and CEO of Wellcoaches Corporation, she has been at the forefront of efforts to establish national standards for professional coaches in health care and wellness since 2000. Moore's team has trained ten thousand health professionals as coaches, who have in turn coached hundreds of thousands of clients seeking to improve their health and their lives.

"My mission in life," she often tells audiences, "is to help people thrive."

Coach Meg is an expert in facilitating change, particularly when change is hard, and in helping people make the kinds of changes that enable them to thrive. As you read these pages, think of her as your personal coach, the one guiding you through the steps that can help transform your survival-mode existence into a thriving, productive, and happy life.

Coauthor Dr. Edward Phillips is the founder and director of the Institute of Lifestyle Medicine at Spaulding Rehabilitation Hospital and is assistant professor of physical medicine and rehabilitation at Harvard Medical School. Dr. Phillips is chair of the Education Committee for the Exercise is Medicine global campaign and is on the board of advisers of the American College of Lifestyle Medicine. He and the Institute of Lifestyle Medicine have been the distinguished recipients of community leadership awards from the President's Council on Physical Fitness, Sports & Nutrition.

While this is not a health and fitness book, per se, lifestyle is important for both physical and mental health. Many individuals who are able to bust stress, tame their frenzy, and flourish actively engage in a healthy lifestyle. Dr. Phillips, known to his patients as Dr. Eddie, has seen firsthand the benefits that accrue when people start and stick with an exercise program, adopt a healthy diet, and do the grueling work necessary to rehab from an injury or illness.

"My greatest satisfaction," he says, "comes from guiding my patients to health and vitality regardless of their present condition."

Dr. Eddie's experiences in helping people along the road to optimum health have informed and enhanced the insights and prescriptions in this book.

Our third coauthor is award-winning writer John Hanc, the author of fourteen books, including Coach Meg's previous book, the bestselling *Organize Your Mind, Organize Your Life*.

This is the team that will provide you with the blueprint to help you tame the frenzy, realize your full capabilities, and thrive. We will do so by teaching you how to listen to yourself better, in order to assess what your needs are and, in turn, figure out what's holding you back.

But we first need to delve into a new theory in psychology, one that deals specifically with human emotions and how they have evolved.

LISTEN TO THE VOICES

Over the course of evolutionary history, our human ancestors developed a set of innate needs, drives, values, capacities, and strengths. These were probably important to survival from primordial times onward, and they have never left us. Recently, they have been shown by scientists to be important factors in generating well-being and peak functioning.

Somewhere along the evolutionary line, these aspects of our personalities likely emerged as *differentiated entities*, also described as *subpersonalities*. These differentiated entities have agendas, which emerge as distinct emotional states and voices. Yes, that's right. Voices. Let's be clear here. We're not likening you to deranged serial killers who claim to have heard voices urging them on as they committed their crimes. That is the stuff of crime novels and TV dramas. What we are saying is that the ongoing inner monologue of our mind is really a dialogue among these differentiated entities. They are multiple aspects of a single personality.

This is not a new idea in psychology. Sigmund Freud, the originator of psychoanalysis, conceptualized the psyche as being divided into an ego, a superego, and an id, each one representing different aspects of our personality, different needs, and different drives.

Over the past twenty-five years, psychologist Richard Schwartz has explored the concept of inner dialogues conducted between the different parts of our psyche. Therapists trained in his Internal Family Systems model of psychotherapy help people invite those parts of themselves—those differentiated entities or subpersonalities of our psyches—that are experiencing negative emotions to a mindful, meditation-like sit-down. These sessions typically follow a winding trail to uncover and heal the small or large traumas experienced by any of the psyche's subpersonalities.

What exactly are these differentiated entities of the psyche, these subpersonalities? Neuroscientists would probably not even consider them as such, but rather as neural networks within the brain that interact with each other. Psychologist John Mayer's landmark personality psychology framework, known as the Systems Framework for Personality Psychology, published in 1995, proposes that each of these differentiated entities, or "agencies," as he calls them, integrates the basic components of our overall personality: emotions, cognitions, behaviors, and consciousness. In other words, our individual traits, what we feel, what we think, and who we think we are may all be encompassed within these differentiated entities of the psyche, these subpersonalities. One might imagine that the brain has a set of neural networks developed and deployed by each of these entities. One of the aims of future research, once more and more people get better at differentiating and addressing these separate entities of the mind and brain, should be to enrich our understanding of the nature and function of these neural networks.

The key to navigating your life and thriving right now is to learn how to discern and tune in to your psyche's differentiated entities, sometimes called the "multiplicity" of your mind— meaning that these multiple subpersonalities play an important role. Emotions can be viewed as important biological messengers sent by these subpersonalities of our psyche. We often think of emotions as handicaps, as barriers to our success. Thus we might say, "Why do I always get so emotional when my father criticizes me? I wish I could stand up to him." Or we might admit, "My anger is keeping me from reaching my goals. I have to learn to control it." Negative emotions are messages alerting us that certain needs are not being met. Conversely, positive emotions tell us that certain needs are being met. Essentially, these emotions serve as a self-management tool, a self-regulatory system that signals our needs in our quest for self-preservation and self-development.

This, by the way, is exactly what eleven-year-old Riley Andersen experiences in the 2015 Pixar film *Inside Out,* which brought the concept of multiplicity of mind to the world, although not in so many words. In the film Riley's basic emotions are personified, giving rise to the characters called Anger, Disgust, Fear, Sadness, and Joy, and they debate how best to respond to her family's big move from Minnesota to San Francisco. Decoding the emotional states of each entity provides clues on how best to improve functioning and collaboration, and thereby reduce inner tension, conflict, stress, and "stuckness" (the sense that we are stuck in a rut and are going nowhere).

This book identifies and explores nine primary differentiated entities of the psyche, which are also termed parts, aspects, and capacities. These nine subpersonalities speak differently to each of us, of course, reflecting our unique genetic mix and our singular experiences, both of which have given rise to our unique capabilities and drives. It's reasonable to suggest that these nine subpersonalities reflect some common human needs and that, therefore, they exist in all of us. And all of us have the capacity to tune in to what our entities are saying.

Here are the nine differentiated entities of the psyche. We will examine each of these in upcoming chapters, but you may already recognize some just by their names.

Autonomy
The Body Regulator
Confidence
The Standard Setter
The Curious Adventurer
The Creative
The Executive Manager
The Relational
The Meaning Maker

In addition to these nine subpersonalities of the psyche, what we like to refer to as the nine members of the Inner Family, there's a tenth aspect that you should know about, the Mindful Self.

Think of it as the one that helps you to hear the others more clearly. The Mindful Self, a concept based upon psychologist Richard Schwartz's model of self-leadership, is the part of the mind that can both discern the nine subpersonalities, those distinct and varied voices, and integrate them to form who we are in a given moment. We will examine the Mindful Self in depth in the next chapter. But it's important to know a little bit about it beforehand, to give you a better understanding of this concept.

The Mindful Self is able to stand back from the Inner Family members and observe, listen to, and discern each of their distinct agendas, capacities, and emotional states. The Mindful Self observes with curiosity, open-mindedness, appreciation, acceptance, and compassion—that is, without judgment. Think of it as that senior manager in the conference room during a heated discussion, the one who listens patiently to all expressed views in the passionate debate and then manages to silence everyone with a clear-as-day comment or a suggestion or observation that cuts to the chase and brings the whole issue into focus.

The Mindful Self is that leader, the conductor of the Inner Family's performance in daily life, encouraging teamwork and harmonious interaction. Ideally, over a lifetime, each Inner Family member (entity or subpersonality) becomes whole, happy, and healthy, having had its needs fully met and having manifested its full potential within the whole self. A person whose Inner Family members are satisfied for the most part, and whose inner capabilities are being harnessed and aligned with inner values, is a person who is *thriving*.

Learning how to tune in to all members of your Inner Family, and to discern what they're telling you, and then recognizing how to act accordingly will enable you to thrive. In this book we will show you how to do that. We will introduce you to each of the members of your Inner Family, and we'll show you how to tune in to what they're saying, so that you can see which of your needs are going unmet and then figure out how to address this in order to achieve balance, improve your overall well-being, and flourish.

Your Inner Family is like your real family in this sense. When someone in your family is unhappy, everyone is affected, and no one can really do their best. When everyone in the family is happy, the family's functioning improves, and the family is imbued with a sense of overall well-being.

We will also show you by example. Coach Meg has taken many of her clients through the process of discerning and acknowledging their Inner Family members. Let's meet two of those clients and see how the subpersonalities, the differentiated entities of the psyche, exert themselves in both positive and negative ways—and how making sense of them, guiding them, and improving their functioning can help you thrive.

NANCY:
After Anger and Defeat, Reason and Success

Nancy came to Coach Meg with an issue that coaches in the health and wellness field commonly address: weight loss. Coach Meg approached the issue of weight loss by first inviting Nancy to tune in to her Inner Family. Coach Meg helped her to recognize the distinct voices of her ongoing internal dialogue, and together they identified three negative emotions: anger, defeat, and frustration.

The anger came from the first voice Nancy heard, that of a harsh inner critic, the Standard Setter, a member of the Inner

Family. "You're a loser," it told her. "You're fat, and you'll always be fat, no matter what you do."

The constant negativity of this inner critic wore down Nancy's Confidence, another member of the Inner Family. The belief in your abilities—or self-efficacy, as psychologists and behavioral theorists call it—is essential to the ability to make meaningful changes. You have to believe that you can do it. Maybe not all of it, and maybe not tomorrow, but at some point. Nancy didn't believe. Her Confidence was shot, in large part because of the constant haranguing by her inner critic. And so she experienced that second emotion she and Coach Meg identified: defeat.

"Why bother?" was what the Standard Setter told Nancy every time she thought about going to the gym or undertaking the effort to prepare a healthy meal. "It's not going to work. We've tried a million diets. We've started and stopped exercising a million times. It's useless."

The third voice that Nancy and Coach Meg were able to tune in to regarding Nancy's weight loss was laced with frustration, the third emotion they pinpointed. This was the voice of what we call the Body Regulator. This is a wise voice that speaks for physiological needs, and it knew full well what Nancy needed to do to incorporate greater physical activity into her life and cut back on unhealthy foods.

By making a few adjustments in her work schedule, she could walk for thirty minutes on her treadmill three times a week and catch an indoor cycling class at the local gym twice a week. This would have been an excellent fitness program, if she had just done it. The Body Regulator also knew that vegetables and fruits are the cornerstone of any successful and healthy diet. There were lots of delicious ways Nancy could begin to eat better.

The Body Regulator was trying to tell Nancy to "eat the apple, not the brownie," to turn off the TV, and to set the alarm clock a half hour earlier so that she could get a walk in before breakfast the following morning. The problem was that this voice was not being listened to. The inner din created by the harsh, angry Standard Setter and defeated Confidence drowned out the wise voice of the Body Regulator. "If you guys can calm down," it was telling her, "I can tell you what to do. You guys are caught up in anger and defeat. But I'm not being listened to."

Just a quick aside here: When we talk about what these voices, that is, these entities or subpersonalities, are saying in this case study and others, we're obviously not referring to verbatim dialogue that has been recorded. "There is a constant stream of inner talk in all our minds," says Coach Meg. "I can tell you from doing hundreds of these sessions that very often the voices we are presenting here are pretty close to the actual dialogue inside."

You will find this to be the case, too, as we go through the process of tuning in to your Inner Family. These interior dialogues are not abstract ruminations from the beyond or some strange psychological phenomenon. They are simply parts of *you* talking to other parts of *you*!

For Nancy, the voice of the Standard Setter needed to be attended to. When she was able to understand what this voice was saying—by using her Mindful Self to observe the competing voices and emotions within her—she came to a couple of realizations.

Coach Meg helped her through that process, which entailed first acknowledging that while its commentary may often be acerbic and even hurtful, the Standard Setter's intentions are good. It sets the bar for achievement and helps establish goals and evaluate progress. It is this capacity that drives us to perform better in our lives. But Nancy had to learn how to change the Standard Setter from an impossible-to-please critic to more of a cheerleader. She realized that this entailed tempering her goals, making them a little more realistic, so as not to disappoint that inner critic. Like many people, Nancy wanted to lose a considerable amount of weight right away. When the results weren't coming as fast as she hoped, the Standard Setter was not happy, and Nancy fell off the wagon. But once she recognized that she had to take some of the pressure off the Standard Setter *and* tuned in to all the messages from members of her Inner Family, she realized that gradual progress was the way to go.

The result? She began to follow the Body Regulator's suggestions about exercise and nutrition. She gradually began to modify her diet; she gradually began to increase her physical activity. Slowly but surely, she began to notice the scale ticking downward. Her confidence rose; she became more upbeat. Small steps, small successes fueled Nancy's determination to stay on track. The Standard Setter's reviews of her performance improved. The Body Regulator did its job. They all worked together toward the same end.

To date, Nancy has lost thirty pounds and has kept it off. She's thriving. She is very proud of her Inner Family!

IAN:
Creating Problems, Organizing Solutions

Ian, a thirty-five-year-old software developer, was a very creative guy. He designed video games of the fantasy, sword, and sorcery variety. As Coach Meg says, "Although I may not be his target audience, I certainly respect what it takes to envision and create these imagined worlds and their various scenarios."

When Meg met him, Ian was also a new father. So like many new moms and dads, he was juggling the demands of being a parent and his career. But there was a particular wrinkle to Ian's situation, which was what compelled him to seek out Coach Meg's help. He had always been disorganized. This is not uncommon among creative people. It's almost a cliché, in fact. But the lack of sleep he was facing as a new father, and the responsibilities a child brought to his life, compounded Ian's disorganization problem.

Ian was missing appointments left and right, was showing up late, and was not responding to e-mails. Once he even double-booked an appointment with a potential new hire and an important client. So he had two people sitting in his waiting room, waiting to meet with him at the same time! This was more than embarrassing. At work, his unreliability was getting beyond the point where his colleagues could just shake their heads, laugh, and say, "Well, that's Ian." He was letting a lot of people down, including his wife. She and the baby were affected, too. For instance, once he forgot to come home to care for the baby when she had a doctor's appointment. And he was angry at himself over all this, although he couldn't seem to get a handle on it.

That was the external picture. Meg discovered after having Ian tune in to his Inner Family that his Creative—not surprisingly, one of his strongest voices—was holding sway, as it always did. It loved spontaneity and disliked structure and any time spent organizing boring stuff. But its powerful voice was now drowning out the one Ian needed to hear the most—that of the Executive Manager. As its name suggests, this is the entity or subpersonality that calls for order.

In one of their sessions, as Coach Meg got Ian to allow his

Executive Manager to articulate its needs, Ian actually stood up and crossed his arms in annoyance.

"What is this voice saying?" Coach Meg asked.

"I don't even know why you bother having me around," Ian responded. "I make lists, I check the schedules, I tell people that I will be there at a certain time, and you just blow me off."

Again, we must interject that the process of tuning in to your inner voices isn't like going into a trance. It's not like something you'd see in a bad made-for-TV movie. Remember that these voices, these emotions, are close to the surface and speak to you constantly. The trick is to discern who is saying what. It's still you, of course, but just a certain part of you.

Coach Meg was able to help Ian discern that his Executive Manager had felt stymied for a long time. But with the increased outside pressures in Ian's life now, the Executive Manager's role was more critical than ever before. Since the Executive Manager was still being ignored, the more things seemed to go awry, the angrier it got.

Once Ian began to understand where his anger was coming from, once he realized that he had this side of himself that could help him try to put some structure and discipline back into his life, he began to ask his Creative to step aside—even when it grumbled, "This is boring!"—and let his Executive Manager do its job, albeit not for too long at a time.

At Coach Meg's suggestion, he scheduled two ten-minute sessions with himself each day—one in the morning, one after lunch—in which he'd essentially recalibrate his day. He would update his to-do list, check his e-mails, and double-check his calendar to make sure he was on top of his commitments.

With these twice-daily organization breaks, Ian was now

giving his Executive Manager an opportunity to be heard and to contribute. And as the Executive Manager began to help him get his life in better order—without sacrificing Creative's wishes—Ian began to appreciate its role.

Is he now an unfailingly punctual person with the neatest desk in the office? No, of course not. He's still Ian, a talented person with a powerful creative drive. But he no longer misses meetings, no longer takes weeks to respond to e-mails, and has allowed at least the outlines of structure to be drawn into his life. Most importantly, he has learned that he has the capacity to manage that part of himself. He just had to listen.

WHAT OUR TEAM CAN DO FOR YOUR TEAM

You want to tame the frenzy and thrive in every aspect of your life. By recognizing that you have at least nine distinct parts to your personality—what we've called entities, subpersonalities, and voices—expressing your primary drives, capabilities, and needs, as well as the Mindful Self, which allows you to better observe these subpersonalities, you can form a clearer picture of how you are conducting your life, and what's at the root of your inner conflicts and ambivalence. Or, as we often say, your "mixed feelings." By listening to what these subpersonalities are saying, and by discerning how they may be driving your behavior in various ways, you can adapt, adjust, and improve the way you do things. In the following chapters we will show you how to do that and more. Here, specifically, are some of the things you will discover from this book:

◆ **You will learn how to pull together as a team:** Your Mindful Self is capable of conducting the orchestra of voices within you, rather than allowing some voices—such as Nancy's Standard Setter or Ian's Creative—to dominate or hijack your brain. When your Inner Family conducts itself as a *team*, its members will be working together toward a common goal—helping *you* thrive in life.

◆ **You will decode the language of your emotions:** We each deal with a frenzied mix of emotions that are constantly changing and are difficult to decode. The voices we do listen to contradict or conflict with each other, leaving us confused about which way to go. If we can link these voices to our emotions and understand what these emotions represent, we can coach ourselves to bring our voices, our Inner Family, into more harmony.

◆ **You will discover strengths you never thought you had:** We often come to misguided conclusions about our strengths and weaknesses. For example, as was the case with Ian, we might think that a disorganized mind is simply an out-of-control Creative, rather than a neglected Executive Manager who is just waiting to be called upon. Conversely, some of us with a highly regulated and organized mind—a mind where the Executive Manager is firmly in control—believe we are not creative and thus limit ourselves. But if we were to modulate the overregulating voice—voilà!—the Creative would speak up. You may not be Van Gogh or Bach, but you can be spontaneous, you can think in a nonlinear way, and you have the ability to think about things in fresh, innovative ways that you never realized.

◆ **You will achieve self-mastery:** This book is a guide you can use to begin to understand what's going on "in there," that is, to make sense of the seeming cacophony of your inner voices. You may have heard the expression "Life is a team sport." When you conceptualize that team as being the various emotions and needs in your head, those differentiated entities of your psyche, all of which must pull together, it's a lot easier to see how to get where you want to go—to a healthier, happier life, to a place where you will thrive. Are you ready? Let's get started!

1

THE NINE MEMBERS OF YOUR INNER FAMILY—AND ONE MINDFUL SELF

People often come to Coach Meg for help when they're struggling. Such was the case not long ago, when a new client made an appointment to discuss her dilemma.

Karen was a single mom with two kids. She needed to get back to work to supplement the child-support payments she was getting from her ex-husband. Karen was well educated—she had a degree in finance and had accrued solid work experience before she became a parent. But when she first visited Coach Meg, it had already been a few years since she left her last job to become a full-time mom. Part of her (the part we call Autonomy) was eager to get back into the corporate world, to show what she was capable of, and to be more self-reliant, so that she didn't have to depend solely on her ex-husband for support. But her Relational capacity—what you might call her "mothering instinct"—was holding her back. She wanted to be available to her kids.

The two subpersonalities she was grappling with, Autonomy and Relational, were both forceful, and they made good points in the internal dialogue that filled her head each day. They even managed to sabotage each other. The nurturing Relational entity asserted itself when Karen wanted to start taking concrete steps toward job hunting. "You can't schedule an appointment with that career counselor today," it would say. "You'll miss David's soccer practice . . . and Jennifer has dance class later. You need to be there for them."

Meanwhile, Autonomy chastised her every time she had to pay a bill or put off a vacation because she was worried about money. "You can do better than this. You don't need to be hand-cuffed by your ex-husband's money, which he is sending you only under duress, anyway. Get out there, and show everyone what you can do on your own."

Coaches have a phrase for the state Karen was in: "Stuck in the muck." Karen was indeed stuck. Two parts of her personality were locked in a stalemate. Her Relational capacity was so strong, it made her drag her feet and prevented her from doing the things she needed to do in order to find a corporate finance position. It was always making excuses. Meanwhile, her drive for Autonomy exhorted her to be true to herself and her talents, and reminded her every day of her dependence on her ex-husband.

For Karen, it was like being caught in the middle of a shouting match; she could no longer hear or think clearly amid the din. And so she was at a standstill, unable to make a move either way. That's the nature of "stuckness," and that's what brought Karen to Coach Meg for help.

After listening carefully to Karen's story, Meg explained the forces within her that were creating the stuckness. She told Karen to try to appreciate that each voice was making a valid point. "After all," Coach Meg said, "these parts, these voices, these members of your Inner Family, are each components of who you are. They are not viruses or some kind of sinister outside influence. This is *you*—or to be more specific, a part of you."

Coach Meg explained that even if it seemed like these voices were at odds with each other, they were each making important points. It was absolutely right that Karen's Relational was driving her to take care of her children; it was equally correct that her Autonomy (backed up her Standard Setter, yet another voice that had joined the fray) wanted her to get to work and to prove to herself and others once again that she was a capable, intelligent, and independent woman.

Coach Meg helped Karen better tune in to and appreciate these voices by asking her to imagine that she could tune in to her mind, in to her subpersonalities, like channels on a radio. She then asked Karen to turn the dial and land on each of these subpersonalities, these voices. Some of Karen's voices came in faintly, as if they originated from a station transmitting from some far-off location. But a couple of them came in with fifty-thousand-watt clarity. They were so loud, in fact, that she almost needed to turn down the volume. It was no surprise which voices were dominating, which came in loud and clear, even if to Karen, they at first sounded like one.

The process of tuning in to your subpersonalities is not one that involves squelching or disconnecting one and amplifying or isolating another. It's usually a process of considering what they all have to say and finding a pathway from there. In other words, we decode the messages our subpersonalities send us by considering how they connect to a set of primary needs, drives, and capacities. Coach Meg shared this approach with Karen. It is this same novel approach that this book offers. (We will learn more about Karen's progress later in this chapter.)

While we all have these nine members of the Inner Family, each of us also has a unique genetic profile mixed with a unique set of experiences that determine and sculpt these entities. Hence there is huge diversity in the Inner Family dynamic.

Given that the nine entities send their messages via our emotional states, we experience a complex and ever-changing mix of feelings. Some emotions are positive, some are negative. Some are subtle, some are loud. What you will learn to do in this book is what Karen and many of Coach Meg's clients have learned to do: translate the language of your emotions into insights on your unique set of needs, drives, capacities, and values—your particular recipe for thriving.

You learned the names of the nine differentiated entities of the psyche, what we like to refer to as the nine members of the Inner Family, in the introduction, and you got a sense of how they influence our behavior in the case studies there. Now it's time to get to know them, to hear what they sound like, and even get a mental picture of how they look!

MEET THE INNER FAMILY

These nine entities of the psyche are expressions of your primary needs, drives, capacities, and values. Together they form the foundation of your personality.

To help you better understand and recognize these different entities, we briefly describe each of them here.

Autonomy

We have a primary need to be the author of our own lives, to engage in the activities that we choose and that reflect our personal values. We dislike external control and can even be rebellious and resistant when we perceive that someone is telling us what we "should" or "have to" do. Conversely, when we have the ability to make a choice, to select something that we find interesting or valuable, we continue to express our autonomy for the sake of it. Autonomy can manifest itself as the drive to leave the nest, to march to our own drummer. Psychologists Edward Deci and Richard Ryan, who have done more than thirty years of research on autonomy, view it as the most primary entity of the human psyche and believe that everything else stems from it.

What Autonomy sounds like:

"I'm not my parents, and I want to do things my way."

"I'm tired of taking orders from someone else. Maybe I should just take a few weeks off, jump on a motorcycle, and drive across the country. Or maybe I'll start my own business."

"I don't want my whole life to revolve around the needs of the others in my family. I want to have a career. I want to pursue my hobbies. I want to march to my own drummer."

What Autonomy looks like:

A woman wearing a stylish leather jacket and skinny leather jeans who drives a sports car.

A twenty-one-year-old man who decides to work in marketing for an up-and-coming local craft brewery, despite the urging of his physician parents to pursue a career in law or medicine.

The Body Regulator

We need equilibrium in all our physiological systems. We seek to balance exertion with resting and recharging. We strive for safety, security, and stability. We listen to our body's signals that tell us when it's time to calm the nervous system, which calms the mind and improves brain function. The Body Regulator is the part of us that knows what our body needs. When you read advice about how to start or stick with an exercise program, and you're urged to "listen to your body," this is the voice you listen to.

What the Body Regulator sounds like:

"Put down that brownie. Your brain will crash after a large jolt of sugar."

"Try to get to bed early tonight. You could use the sleep."

"Take a break this weekend. You've been working really hard, and you don't want to burn out or get sick."

What the Body Regulator looks like:

- A fit, trim yoga instructor who not only understands what it takes to be healthy, but is also a master of balance, literally and figuratively, which is what the Body Regulator is all about.
- A trim seventy-year-old man who takes indoor cycling classes at the gym, works with a personal trainer, and maintains a healthy diet in order to manage the type 1 diabetes that he has had since childhood.

Confidence

We have a basic need to be confident and competent. This is the "lion" in all of us, an entity that is sometimes proud and almost regal in its bearing, and sometimes too much (if there is an overabundance of this quality). Our sense of strength or empowerment is a key determinant of our actions. If we don't believe we can do something, we are less likely to try it. It's not uncommon to have tension between Confidence and the Standard Setter, our judging voice, the part of us that has a measuring stick and sets the bar, perhaps too high.

What Confidence sounds like:

- "I can repair this broken faucet."
- "I can make this relationship work."
- "I can finish this project on deadline, when the boss needs it. No problem."

What Confidence looks like:

A skilled, sure-handed manager who strides the office floor, solving problems presented to her, issuing orders, and inspiring employees, confident in her ability to manage a workplace that hums with efficiency.

A forty-year-old entrepreneur in jeans and a blazer who is as eager to tell you about the high-tech ventures he's launched that have failed as he is about the ones that have succeeded. (He will tell you this, by the way, while he takes you for a ride in his expensive sports car, and he'll suggest that what he learned from his failures helped fuel his successes.)

The Standard Setter

This part of us carries a measuring stick, sets the bar or standard, and judges and evaluates how well we are performing in life, both in terms of what we think about our own performance and how others evaluate and value our contributions. The Standard Setter judges our performance across all domains of life. It is highly active in the social realm, since we are social beings who seek approval, appreciation, validation, and fair treatment. This is a fundamental necessity for humans, the most social animals on the planet. No man is an island. We want to be accepted and appreciated by our peers, our friends and family, our community.

At its worst, this entity of our psyche is difficult to please. The Standard Setter can be an inner critic, scanning for flaws and faults, or ever raising the bar to unattainable levels. At its best, it is accepting and content, setting challenging goals, while adopting a learning or growth mind-set, focused on "What am I learning, and how am I getting better?" when performance falls short.

What the Standard Setter sounds like:

"You didn't get this done."
"You should have told your sister-in-law to mind her own
    business."
"You really messed up on that assignment."

or

"You really did a good job on this."
"Hey, mistakes happen. We'll learn from that."
"You should feel good about what you did at work today."

What the Standard Setter looks like:

A judge, with a gown and a gavel, who could be either a
    compassionate, lenient judge (and would give you a
    suspended sentence) or a hanging judge.
A fifty-five-year-old woman who stays in shape through
    walking and yoga classes, but has let go of the need to
    have the physique of a thirty-year-old.

The Curious Adventurer

The need to experience novel situations, to explore, learn, and change is what compels humans to climb mountains and conquer new frontiers. In his book *Curious?: Discover the Missing Ingredient to a Fulfilling Life*, psychologist Todd Kashdan asserts that curiosity is a primary driver of human well-being, saying, "Curious explorers are comfortable with the risks of taking on new challenges. . . . Instead of trying desperately to explain and control our world, as a curious explorer we embrace uncertainty . . . and see our lives as an enjoyable quest to discover, learn, and grow." In the rapidly transforming world of the early twenty-first century, this is a highly relevant capacity, as our ability to embrace change is part of what can help us succeed in the new economy. But of course, it doesn't necessarily have to apply only to the big things in life, as the name of this entity may suggest.

What the Curious Adventurer sounds like:

"I'm tired of eating the same old thing for dinner. Let's go get Ethiopian tonight."
"I'm bored with the same old, same old holiday routine. Let's go celebrate Christmas in the Caribbean."
"I think it's time for me to buy a new computer. I've been PC for years. Maybe it's time for a Mac."

What the Curious Adventurer looks like:

A young woman with a backpack who is on her way to explore a remote mountain for the first time.
A couple who have decided to go on a historical walking tour of the city they've lived in for years.

The Creative

We have a basic need to be creative, generative, imaginative, and spontaneous. The Creative works best when our minds are unleashed and allowed to wander about, unplugged from deadlines and goals. This part of us has fun brainstorming, playing games, and being impulsive. When in full action, it produces flow states, those moments where we are enjoying an activity so much that we lose track of time as we're doing it.

What the Creative sounds like:

> "I've got an idea for a new way to organize my e-mails."
> "I want to try a different exercise routine in the gym, using just my body weight as resistance."
> "I want to come up with a different lesson plan for my students."

What the Creative looks like:

> A chef in the kitchen who has a tableful of ingredients in front of her and an idea for a new pasta dish.
> An investment banker who, when he returns home at night, sheds his three-piece suit for story time with his young daughter, during which time he is happy to act out the various parts—complete with exaggerated pseudo-French accent—in the Madeline series.

The Executive Manager

Thank goodness our brains have a primary need to be organized, to plan, to regulate our emotions and impulses, and to keep us on track. We call this need the Executive Manager, a capable self-regulator who sets aside disruptive emotions, impulses, and distractions because of its strong desire to be productive.

What the Executive Manager sounds like:

"Let's check the to-do list for today."
"Have you scheduled your annual checkup with the doctor?"
"Do we have everything packed for the trip?"
"Are we shopping for the healthy foods we need to be eating?"

What the Executive Manager looks like:

An accountant who has gotten all the tax forms ready for his clients by April 15.

A parent who has food in the fridge, has the laundry done, and has a clean house.

An administrative assistant who keeps his boss's calendar and commitments organized and helps the organization run with clockwork efficiency.

The Relational

We all want to love and be loved by others, to serve others, to help others get their needs met, and to feel we belong. The entity of the psyche at work here is what we term the Relational. It is the voice of compassion within us, our compassion for others and our *self*-compassion. It is essential for taming and calming our inner frenzy and our negative emotions.

The Relational can conflict with our need for autonomy and adventure. Throughout life, we must balance our desire to do our own thing and to pursue novel experiences with our need for relationships. There are times when maintaining this balance demands many adjustments, such as when we choose to get married or have children.

What the Relational sounds like:

> "What can I do to help my son? He's angry over not making the football team, and I want to help make him feel better about it."
>
> "I'm concerned about my friend, who is so upset over things that are happening in her life."
>
> "My colleague lost her husband recently, and I know she's still hurting. Maybe I should send her some flowers or just give her a call and let her know we all miss her at work."

What the Relational looks like:

A parent who is caring.

A generous-hearted, supportive coach who cares about his players and gets the most out of everyone on the team by bringing out their best.

A boss who mentors her staff.

The Meaning Maker

We have a primary need to pose the big questions of what it means to be human, to find meaning and purpose in our lives, whether it's in the daily tasks we perform or in the grand scheme of things, of which we are all a part. We are hardwired to seek a higher purpose for our lives, to grow beyond our self-interest, to ponder the big picture of our existence, to try to figure out our place within the universe. This is the realm of the Meaning Maker.

What the Meaning Maker sounds like:

"Why am I having such a hard time with my relationship?"

"How does what I do in my job change anything for the better?"

"I think I was meant to be with this person."

"Why is there so much misery and violence in the world?"

What the Meaning Maker looks like:

Henry David Thoreau in his cabin in the woods.
A woman at the beach who is staring out at the vastness of the ocean.
Family members who have their heads bowed at their place of worship.
A college student who has in hand a book on the ancient Greek philosophers.

We'll look more closely at the nine members of the Inner Family, the Inner Tribe, in later chapters. But before we zoom in, we need to pan back. Our minds have the capacity to detach from our noisy inner voices and emotions, to experience the action in our brains as if we are watching a movie. This natural brain state, called meta-awareness or, more commonly, mindfulness, is critical for self-reflection and change. It allows us to be less reactive to passing emotional states and enables us instead to observe, identify, and accept them without feeling hijacked and out of control. When we are in a mindful, open state, we can be curious about decoding our emotional status, rather than getting caught up in the frenzy. So mindfulness is a home base of sorts, this default that gives us perspective, allows us to see with greater objectivity our various needs and ourselves.

In this book we like to refer to mindfulness, or meta-awareness, as the Mindful Self. We characterized it in the introduction as the conductor of the Inner Family's performance in daily life, fostering collaboration and harmonious interaction. Gaining an understanding of the Mindful Self is the first step toward being able to discern and decode our other needs. It is the place where we begin our journey to self-discovery, where we set off down the road to a life in which we are truly flourishing.

THE MINDFUL SELF

"Who are you?" sang the eponymously named rock band The Who in one of their biggest hits of the 1970s. It's a question we all ask at one time or another. Some spend a lifetime searching for a meaningful answer; some go through years of therapy, climb mountains, take drugs, or remove themselves to remote, exotic locations in search, supposedly, of this elusive definition of *self*.

In terms of what we're talking about in this book, the "who" that you are is composed of those various subpersonalities, those entities of the psyche, that express various drives and needs common to us all.

But overarching these is what we call the Mindful Self. Understanding what that is and the role it plays is a critical first step to being able to tune in to those various subpersonalities, in order to ultimately bring them into harmony.

What does the term *Mindful Self* mean? Psychologist Richard Schwartz, the creator of the Internal Family Systems model of psychotherapy, has studied self-leadership for twenty-five years. He defines the *self* as "the core of a person," embodying qualities such as compassion, clarity, curiosity, and confidence. It is the self, Schwartz says, that is best equipped to lead the Inner Family—the nine subpersonalities. The "mindful" part refers to the ability of the self to stand back from the Inner Family, to observe, listen to, and discern each distinct agenda, capacity, or emotion with curiosity, open-mindedness, and compassion—and, very importantly, without judgment.

You've met those other members of the tribe, those subpersonalities. Schwartz likes to conceptualize the Mindful Self as the *self* leader, as the conductor of that internal orchestra whose members are your subpersonalities. You can almost imagine him or her, in tails or a black tux or a formal gown, stepping onto the stage and taking the podium. Aside from the tapping of his baton, he makes no noise. He doesn't play an instrument. He is simply conducting. Amid the nonstop dialogue that goes on in all our minds, it is that internal conductor, the Mindful Self, who can help create order out of what may seem like the chaotic, dissonant interplay of our various subpersonalities.

Like a conductor attending to each section of the orchestra and each instrument on the stage, the Mindful Self is able not only to listen to the voices that are a part of your personality and synthesize them, but also to discern their separateness, their independent agendas. That's important. It allows us to zero in on and then detach from our negative emotions. The Mindful Self says, "There's a part of me that's upset, but it's only *part* of me. It's not all of me. There's another part of me that's probably not upset, but I have been so focused on the part that is upset, that I didn't realize that until now."

The Mindful Self is a core feature of your mind that can help you keep things in perspective and prevent one dominant voice, especially a negative one, from overwhelming every aspect of your life. It's those negative voices that cause the feeling of frenzy, and that's what mindfulness can help prevent or mitigate. An example: You get angry at your spouse. Let's say that the part that's angry is Confidence, because your spouse hasn't shown much of it in you. He or she has been a bit snarky lately, making comments about how you're incapable of doing this or that—or at least that's how you hear it. Now, your Confidence, which is taking a hit, is talking up a storm, saying nasty things and getting you in trouble. The Mindful Self observes the uncoiling anger. "Uh-oh," it might say. "My blood pressure is rising, and my face is turning red. Part of me is very angry. Oh, I feel this. It's a sign that there's something wrong, I need to pay attention to it. But maybe I should go for a walk and not yell at my spouse, even though I am hurt by his [or her] lack of confidence in me." (We use this same story later.)

As you can see, the Mindful Self is calm, cool, open, reflective, measured, nonjudgmental, and patient. The Mindful Self recognizes and helps soothe the angry voice (and, again, remember such voices are generally an expression of specific and unmet needs, so they should be heeded), and it also expresses appreciation and gratitude for the positive contributions that each member of the Inner Family is making. It is the Mindful Self that can channel compassion and alleviate any negative emotions and suffering. It is the Mindful Self that helps a member of the Inner Family get its needs met and then capitalizes on that member's abilities.

But we shouldn't confuse orchestration with action. The Mindful Self itself is not the creator, the motivator, or the confident leader who rallies the troops together and yells, "Charge!" There are other members of your Inner Family that have the capacity to perform those functions. The Mindful Self integrates all those capacities into the daily melody and harmony of life. Being mindful is about *being in the moment,* experiencing and observing, integrating and conducting.

That's a gentle call to action that you may have heard before, especially if you've ever taken a meditation or yoga class. That command is, "Focus on your breath in the now, in the moment." The instructor invites you to be aware of your breathing, to observe it, to experience it. You are encouraged to neither live in the past nor anticipate the future. You are gently urged to put aside your to-do list and forget about the annoying phone call or meeting this morning.

But you don't necessarily have to sit cross-legged on the floor and focus on your breathing in order to be in a state of mindfulness. You can be mindful in the middle of that meeting, or while you're taking a walk or just sitting in your living room. "Mindfulness," said the Zen Buddhist monk and teacher Thich Nhat Hanh at a 2013 Harvard Medical School conference, "has an object. So if you're simply sitting still like a frog, you're mindful of what's going on inside of you and around you, in the present."

That's an important point. When you are mindful, you're not just staring into space or trying to achieve some kind of state of nothingness. You are mindful *of* something. Of breathing or eating or reacting to your boss's feedback. When you're mindful of eating, you're noticing the smells of the food, the different flavors in your mouth, the way your jaw moves, the clatter of the silverware. You're not eating the project that's due tomorrow or chewing on the particulars of the argument you had with your partner last night.

Jon Kabat-Zinn, the founding executive director of the Center for Mindfulness in Medicine, Health Care, and Society at the University of Massachusetts Medical School, has much the same take on mindfulness. He describes mindfulness as being in the present tense, as thinking about life in terms of gerunds—that is, verb forms ending in *-ing:* experiencing, observing, watching.

As we now know from brain imaging, mindfulness occurs deep and low in the brain and more toward the back, the more primitive part of the brain. This is something we share with animals. Indeed, they live continually in the moment. They don't tell stories about what they've seen or worry about the future. When a frog is sitting still, it is just experiencing. There's a book about mindfulness for kids called *Sitting Still Like a Frog*. How appropriate.

If a frog, your dog or cat, and most first graders can learn how to be present, or mindful, so can you. Let's talk about how.

MINDING YOUR OWN MINDFULNESS

Achieving mindfulness doesn't have to entail sitting cross-legged on a mat, eyes closed. You don't need to don the robes of a monk or burn incense. While adherents of such traditions are often very good at achieving the state of mindfulness, this state is accessible to anyone and in all kinds of familiar environments.

Coach Meg begins each morning with a simple mindfulness exercise. "I say to myself, 'I am still. I am here,'" she says. "I am in the 'now,' the present moment. I look around. I notice my living room. I notice how I feel. It takes five to ten seconds. You don't have to do this for hours. You can experience the moment for a few seconds or a few breaths."

Even that brief period of time devoted to mindfulness can have a powerful effect on you, like hitting a reset button. "When you go into deep sensory parts of your brain, you free yourself from narrating, thinking, worrying, pushing. You free yourself from the frenzy," Coach Meg says. "It's a 'no frenzy zone.'"

While mindfulness may seem like something new and unfamiliar, it's not. You've been mindful before; you've experienced this sensation before. We all have. We started our lives being in the moment. Babies don't think about the past, the present, and the future. They have only now. They're aware. They're experiencing all the time. What happens is, as we grow up, our brains just get so cluttered with stuff that we forget how to be mindful. The point of mindfulness exercises, including meditation, is to take us to this place we knew as children, this simple place where we are just experiencing. It's a place of just watching. We're not thinking. We're present and experiencing this place, as opposed to being caught up in thinking about what's happening.

Mindfulness is essential to well-being. It's here, in this state of "now," of mindfulness, that you can tune in to your emotions, your voices, the nine entities of your psyche. They're important. After all, they're running the show; they're your Inner Tribe. There's no music without the voices. However, we're so used to certain voices being in charge, we've lost the ability to step back from them. We've just let them take over. Moreover, we can't even tell them apart sometimes. The challenge we have is to hear all the voices. The Mindful Self is the integration of all our voices at their best. It's calm, cool, open, and measured. It's nonjudgmental and patient.

It's a good place to be.

How do we get there? How do we get to this oasis of mindfulness? Coach Meg teaches people that one way is to imagine that your attention is moving into the deeper sensory recesses of your brain. You're sitting now and reading this book. Your brain is focusing, thinking, absorbing. Your attention shines like a spotlight—almost as if it's emanating from your forehead. But imagine that this spotlight is on wheels. Let's back it up. Now dim the light. Put down the book for a moment. And notice where you are. In this moment. In the now.

You're not living in the front of the brain. Your conscious attention, your spotlight, is deep and low. You're simply *here*.

You can close your eyes or not. Just experience the moment . . . this moment. The sun is shining through the window, or maybe the rain is streaking the windowpane.

Observe your breath. The slight tension in your shoulders. The temperature in the room. A car passes by. . . . You hear it, and you acknowledge it.

Use one sense at a time. What are you seeing as you dispassionately scan the room? What are you hearing? What are you smelling, feeling? The white-hot light of your attention may have been pushed back and put on low for the time being, but you feel that your senses are sharp, even heightened.

Coach Meg views the mindful state as a home base for her. Prior to starting any project or task, she tries to visit home base, to bring herself to that mindful place. Before a conference call, she sits in front of her computer and looks at her phone. She's conscious of the computer, the phone, the messages, but she's not allowing the voices or the stimuli to overwhelm her.

This is the Mindful Self. It's a "sensing and experiencing" mode, as opposed to the place where we are being driven by our narratives, our needs, and our voices (the place where most of us are every day). We have to escape that place where we have to get this done, that done, have to be here, have to be there. We have to step back to look in. Simply by being mindful, even for ten seconds or less, is the way we do that.

Try practicing mindfulness once a day, if possible. You can do it anywhere or anytime. Establishing the home base of mindfulness will enable you to listen better to the members of your Inner Family, the nine subpersonalities who all have something to say to you.

And how might you talk to your nine subpersonalities once you have achieved a mindful state? Psychologist Ethan Kross has studied how best to conduct one's inner dialogue, or self-talk. In his 2011 paper entitled "Boosting Wisdom: Distance from the Self Enhances Wise Reasoning, Attitudes, and Behavior," Kross explains that people need a mechanism to transcend the Velcro-like grip of inner concerns, and that people can easily be taught to view themselves as a "fly on the wall," which leads them to more wisdom and open-mindedness. In a 2015 *Psychology Today* article entitled "The Voice of Reason," Kross notes that by "toggling the way we address the self . . . [that is, either in the] first person or third person . . . we flip a switch in the cerebral cortex, the center of thought, and another in the amygdala, the seat of fear. Using the third person, i.e., this part of me, rather than 'I,' brings psychological distance from negative thoughts and emotions. It enables self-control, allowing us to gain perspective, think more clearly, and perform at our best."

Throughout this book we will show you how to conduct a dialogue with the various subpersonalities in the third person, so that each subpersonality speaks for itself and is spoken to, and is separate from the others and from the Mindful Self. Sounds a little far-fetched? Maybe, but as Kross's research teaches us, this mode of inner dialogue allows us to have a healthy rapport with the various parts of our psyche, improving our self-control and even moving us toward self-mastery. And as you will see in our case studies, such inner conversations and debates are often lively, to say the least, and can go a long way toward helping people resolve issues that have stymied them sometimes for their entire lives. And making this leap will hasten their progress in the journey to thriving.

So now let's learn how to listen and talk to our nine entities of the psyche, our subpersonalities. As you will recall, this is precisely what Coach Meg taught her client Karen, the single mom with two kids who was chomping at the bit to get back into the corporate world but was concerned about the impact that this action would have on her children's well-being.

Over the course of four sessions with Coach Meg, Karen learned—much as you have—about her Inner Family. She came to understand that two members of her Inner Family, her Autonomy and her Relational capacity, were deadlocked over her decision either to return to the workforce or to remain in the home as a full-time mom.

Coach Meg instructed Karen on how to achieve a mindful state, and once Karen mastered that, Coach Meg introduced her to each of the nine subpersonalities and told her to forge a dialogue with each one in the third person to create a little distance. "Hello, Autonomy. What would you like to say about this situation?" Karen began, and then she listened to what Autonomy had to say about her conundrum. Karen addressed each subpersonality in the same way and heard each one out. Interestingly, they were almost split evenly as to whether Karen should rejoin the corporate world or remain in the home:

> *Autonomy* was angry. "Stop wasting time. Step up and do what's needed. Start checking Craigslist, get in touch with your old boss, work your contacts, and set up interviews."
>
> *Confidence* was hesitant. "I can do this . . . but I'm not sure I can command a six-figure salary. I don't know if anyone will hire me for big bucks."
>
> *The Creative* was eager to get going. "Put the tension aside and get on with it. I know I'll be able to come up with some innovative ways of doing things that will help us meet both goals."

The Executive Manager was frustrated. "We're getting sidetracked. We need to get organized here and get going."

The Body Regulator reminded Karen to be consistent with her exercise, not only for her physical health. "You know you always feel better after a vigorous workout. You'll be more focused at work and less stressed out when you get home to the kids."

The Curious Adventurer was intrigued with the idea of returning to the workforce. "A new challenge, in a new environment . . . It's going to be exciting!"

The Standard Setter was critical. "I can't be a good mom and perform at a high level in a job at the same time. So therefore, we should not be going back to work right now."

The Relational was worried about Karen's kids. "They're very sensitive. How are they going to handle you being less available? Autonomy is being very selfish here!"

And *the Meaning Maker* put it all into perspective. "I need both for my well-being. It's vital to support my need for autonomy, as well as nurture my compassionate side."

Think we're making this up? These are almost verbatim comments in Coach Meg's notes from her session with Karen in which Coach Meg encouraged her to tune in to her different subpersonalities and allow them each to give voice to their views on and concerns about the dilemma that had her stuck. "The session with Karen reminded me yet again that these parts are really, truly independent voices," Coach Meg says. "It never ceases to amaze me that each of us has these different perspectives. And yet they can sound as one if you don't know what you're listening for."

In future chapters, you will learn how to discern each of the nine subpersonalities and allow them to express themselves to you, in order to move you out of your "stuckness," your anxieties, or whatever it is that is keeping you from flourishing. But first, you might be wondering, what happened to Karen? Well, after much procrastination, Autonomy finally won out. Karen started looking for a full-time position, and before long she found one as a corporate finance officer. It was a good job, with a substantial salary and a lot of responsibilities. Right up to the night before she started, she still had doubts about reigniting her career. She could still hear her Relational voice expressing fear that her selfish Autonomy would take over, and that she'd get immersed in work and neglect the kids.

She *did* get immersed in work—she had learned that she needed to give her drive for Autonomy more attention—but she also made a conscious effort to remain diligent in her parenting duties. The Executive Manager and the Creative were both happy to figure out new and more efficient ways to organize her time to enable her to do that. And as it turned out, some of Relational's fears were unfounded: Karen's kids, David and Jennifer, were excited about their mom's new job. They thought it was cool that she was entrusted with managing millions of dollars. They also saw that she was happier putting her skills and her education to use, and so they were happier, too.

Karen, we're happy to say, is now unstuck. She has tamed the frenzy that had emerged from her emotional stalemate, and although she's working hard, she is thriving. That's where we're going to guide you, too: first to a mindful state and then to an understanding of how to discern these different voices and, ultimately, orchestrate them so as to achieve more balance and fulfillment. You'll learn how in the next few chapters.

DR. EDDIE:
A Personal Case Study in Mindfulness

Arriving as a freshman on the Yale campus in September 1977, I was eager to learn but was intimidated by the intellectual rigor of the school. I was humbled by the imposing architecture on campus but felt sheltered by the fortresslike edifices from the grittiness of New Haven, just outside Yale's walls. However, after a few short weeks, a workers' strike closed the dining halls and compelled me to venture off the campus in search of breakfast. When I ventured out from the confines of the classroom and the campus, looking for a meal, I did not expect to find my mindfulness mentor dressed in an apron.

I headed to my favorite spot, immediately adjacent to the Old Campus: Claire's Corner Copia—that's a play on the word *cornucopia,* as in a bountiful harvest of diner food. Sitting at the counter, I ordered my eggs and opened my calculus textbook in an effort to remain productive. When the food arrived, I muttered my thanks and dug into my eggs, home fries, and toast, while still focused on a nearly indecipherable problem on a page of my textbook. As I mindlessly took my second bite, Claire herself slammed the textbook closed, causing me and my plate to jump. I looked up sheepishly at the cook, who at this moment was like a mother who had just discovered her son reading a copy of *Playboy* magazine.

"When you eat . . . *eat*! When you read . . . *read*!"

At that moment, I discovered that not all college learning is done in the classroom. But who would have predicted that my first lesson in mindfulness would come not from some Eastern philosophy professor or in a Transcendental Meditation class, but in a local diner, from its gruff but caring owner?

Needless to say, my focus for the rest of the time I was at Claire's that day was on her delicious food. The math problems could wait. The impact of what she said, however, was far-reaching. To this day, as I venture through life, Claire's edict continues to impact on my sensibility and approach to things, while calculus has little, if any, relevance.

I am far from being a cloistered monk leading a meditative life, but over time I have done my best to follow Claire's advice and become more conscious of what I am actively doing, being, and feeling in the moment. I have frankly felt behind the times, as the world seems to have sped up and adopted the mantra of multitasking. I have never mastered the task of searching the Internet, writing an e-mail, and participating in a conference call simultaneously. Any attempt to split my focus leaves me stressed and confused. I was heartened to begin reading studies reporting that humans are not designed to attend fully to more than one stimulus at a time. In fact, I soon realized in the midst of a stressful week of writing deadlines, phone calls, research studies, administrative headaches, and constant interruptions, that my one-on-one time knee to knee with my patients was consistently the most intense, fulfilling, and rejuvenating professional experience of the week. My mindful, concentrated focus and the human connection are critical to my patients feeling heard and are vital to my own health and well-being.

As someone who passionately promotes exercise as foundational to a healthy lifestyle, I sought to increase my own physical activity in the midst of too many commitments and too little time by adopting *multipurpose* tasks, such as walking meetings and watching the news from the saddle of my exercise bicycle. However, I soon realized that more fully conscious exercise, such as yoga, outdoor bicycling (being fully attentive to the road, the traffic, the bicycle, and my exertion), flipping tires in boot camp class, or Zumba (making sure I don't trip over my own two feet), evokes a more peaceful and revitalized feeling than distracted physical activity with a distracted mind.

Years after graduating from Yale, I participated in a seminar with Dr. Jon Kabat-Zinn, the physician who helped popularize the term *mindfulness* through his research and a series of bestselling books. In the course of his presentation, I learned to fully experience texture, smell, and taste as I slowly and consciously chewed and swallowed a single raisin over several minutes. When I chatted with him afterward, I related the story of Claire, my first mindfulness teacher. He listened intently to the brief story and declared, "Pure Zen. And what *chutzpah!*" Indeed, Claire did "get in my face," as my children would say, and it made a difference.

I was devoted to improving my own mindfulness, but at one point I wondered whether I was confronting my patients as best I could to help them become more mindful and healthier. I thought that perhaps I should confront my patients with a more paternalistic imperative to become mindful and relax. I considered the comical scene of me (and so many other expectant fathers) "soothing" their laboring wives in the delivery room, screaming, "Relax!" and "Breathe!" I stepped back and analyzed the stressful first few minutes of an office visit with a new patient. The patient would be anxious to get his or her story across, hopeful for some relief from pain and discomfort. I decided to try to change this paradigm. During the first minute of a visit, as my computer slowly booted up, I had the habit of using the slowly rotating hourglass on the computer screen as a cue to take a long, deep relaxing breath. I had been modeling this mini relaxation exercise, but with my next patient, I took a leap and invited her to breathe with me: "Breathe slowly and effortlessly, in and out through your nose." She did. She visibly calmed, her speech slowed, and her urgency lessened. She was already on her way to understanding the link between her pain and stress.

Thirty-six years after my first meal in New Haven, I returned to the Yale campus, no longer as a student, but as a visiting professor, honored to have been asked to deliver grand rounds at the medical school later that morning. It was quite an honor, but as I would find out that day, one is never too senior or too important to learn life lessons at a luncheonette. Given the opportunity that morning, I headed straight to the renovated Claire's Corner Copia for breakfast. I ordered my meal from the counter and sat down to wait at a table. I asked for Claire and learned that while still in charge of the restaurant, she was off for the day, unfortunately, so I could not share with her how her eight-word imperative had affected my life. Intent on remaining mindful of my eating and honoring her injunction, I put away my cell phone, closed the newspaper, and focused on the remarks I would soon deliver to the Department of Psychiatry.

When my eggs arrived, I reflexively reached for the saltshaker but found none on my table. I turned toward the adjoining table, which was also devoid of salt. I looked around and found that all fifteen saltshakers were neatly lined up on a shelf across the room. Annoyed, I got up from my seat and immediately assessed blame; I assumed the busboy was lax in distributing the shakers to the tables. However, when I was close enough, I read the sign with Claire's words that had been affixed to the shelf:

WHY DO WE KEEP THE SALTSHAKERS HERE? WE WANT TO ENCOURAGE YOU TO TRY OUR FOOD BEFORE ADDING SALT. A LOW-SALT DIET IS PROVEN TO HELP LOWER BLOOD PRESSURE. A HEALTHY LIFESTYLE IS A HAPPY LIFE-STYLE.

The eggs were delicious, without any added salt. I had returned to New Haven, to Claire's Corner Copia, for yet another lesson in mindfulness. Even in absentia, Claire, my mindfulness mentor, had taught me another lesson:

Hold the salt, and savor the moment.

Here are a few additional pieces of advice to help you achieve this state of mindfulness:

1. Designate a frequently occurring event—such as the spinning circle on your computer screen as your computer boots up, or a red light while you are driving—as your cue to take a long, deep breath and become aware of your surroundings and your most prevalent feeling at the time. These frequent mini mindfulness breaks will soon build on each other and become easier.

2. If you have pain or physical discomfort, take a moment to assess your stress level (tune in to the Body Regulator) and then listen to the other eight voices before reflexively reaching for pain medication. You may find that you can get by with less or even forgo the medication altogether.

3. Try not to react immediately to events, comments, and circumstances. Instead, try mentally to "hit the pause button" and allow for a "mindfulness moment." It is the momentary silence between the musical notes that changes an overwhelming cacophony of noise into a soaring musical score. That same second or two can often defuse a stressful situation, not to mention prevent a response you may regret later.

ROLL CALL! WHO'S WHO IN YOUR INNER FAMILY

In her bestselling novel *Divergent,* author Veronica Roth envisions a future in which members of society can be classified into five factions: those who are predominantly selfless, peaceful, honest, brave, or knowledgeable. Roth imagines that once individuals reach the age of sixteen, they must undergo an aptitude test to identify which of the social and personality types they possess and thus which of the factions they will be affiliated with. Those who believe that at birth they clearly belong to one faction or the other demonstrate their traits proudly. For example, the Dauntless (brave) ones jump off moving trains upon their arrival at the "choosing ceremony" to show their courage. "The future belongs to those who know where they belong!" the initiates are told by one official.

The heroine of the series, though, is a "divergent," someone who cannot be pigeonholed into one of the five factions, but rather exhibits personality traits emblematic of several of the factions. This young woman is the one who recognizes what it means to be truly human, and a moral of the book is that few of us can be so driven by a single trait, virtue, or emotion that it comes to define who we are. The fragile balance and tension among the various factions within this future society and within the character herself in the novel is a fine metaphor for the very real, ongoing competition between the nine entities of the psyche, the nine subpersonalities within us, the idea at the heart of the Internal Family Systems model and this book.

These subpersonalities, and the emotions through which they articulate their needs, did not appear overnight. They likely evolved over millions of years. Most of them are not even unique to humans. You probably have never thought of yourself as having much in common with bacteria, among the simplest and most ancient life-forms on Earth, right? You'd be surprised. Humans share 7 percent of their genes with bacteria. Here's one of the physiological processes they have in common: Bacteria, single-celled microorganisms, have pores that open and close based on the conditions around them. If the environment is conducive, these pores open and let in nutrition; if the environment is toxic, the pores close. This is the primitive example of the fulfillment of an organism's basic need for stability, or homeostasis, defined as "the maintenance of metabolic equilibrium within an animal by a tendency to compensate for disrupting changes." Homeostasis is critical to the human animal's survival, too. All the physiological systems in human beings—digestion, circulation, respiration, and so on—are calibrated to maintain balance. There's a rhythm to the flow of blood, the pumping of the heart, the breathing of the lungs, the contraction of our muscles.

Interestingly, the dictionary offers a second definition of

homeostasis: "the maintenance of equilibrium within a social group, person, etc." This means that this need for stability exists beyond the level of the organism and extends to a school, a corporation, a team, an army, or any other organized assemblage of humans.

Homeostasis permeates our higher consciousness and our collective consciousness, as well. One of the oldest and most basic of our needs is the need for security and stability, individually and collectively, and it is this need that drives us to say "Don't." We might tell a friend, "Don't climb Mount Everest." We might tell our children, "Don't venture out into the blizzard." We might tell our spouse, "Don't take that new job or even leave the house." And if we're talking to a group, we might say, "Don't rock the boat."

This is the opposite of risk tasking. This is risk avoidance, and it's as old as the living organisms we evolved from.

In humans, that need for safety, for balance, for homeostasis translates into the subpersonality we call the **Body Regulator**.

Here's where it gets complicated. The next level on the hierarchy of needs, posited by psychologist Abraham Maslow and others, is the need for risk taking: the exact opposite of the need for safety. Bacteria simply open and close their pores to get nutrients or not, as the situation warrants. They do not move about, hunting down nutrients. But more sophisticated organisms need to go out and seek whatever it is they are after. This seeking is a form of risk taking, and it, too, is embedded in our genes. This is the need that likely enabled early humans to hunt game.

As humans evolved, this risk-taking capacity expressed itself in other ways. It compelled us to explore the next valley, the next continent, and the moon. It made us say yes to the idea of trying to summit Mount Everest, even when the more conservative Body Regulator said no.

In our typology, the risk taker, this innovative, adventure-seeking, experimental subpersonality is what we call the **Curious Adventurer**.

Somewhere along the evolutionary continuum, predators—organisms that attack and kill other organisms in order to survive—appeared. What does predation require? A projection of strength and power. Whether it's the baring of teeth, the puffing of frill or feathers, or a deafening roar, predators know how to make themselves look big and strong and how to strike fear into their prey. The predatory drive and the traits associated with it help make the lion the king of the jungle, even though it's not the largest, faster, strongest, or smartest creature. But, boy, the lion is confident, and it knows how to project that self-assuredness.

Humans exhibit these traits, too. Leaders have them in spades. Throughout history, chiefs, kings, queens, and others with commanding authority have known how to carry themselves and project themselves to instill maximum fear and respect among their people. The typical modern-day CEO possesses these traits, too.

This is the subpersonality we call **Confidence**.

When managed successfully, however, this subpersonality is moderated by individuals' knowledge of their own competence and limitations. Successful early hunters probably learned that no amount of name-calling and spear pounding would work against a saber-toothed tiger . . . unless there were many hunters working together. This is an example of the capacity to create communities, groups of people with a common interest who come together. Communities didn't start with humans. Consider the beehive. Here you have a colony with its own complex social hierarchy. In order to fit in and get enough to eat, you, the bee, have to be aware of your role and how well you're doing, or you could be kicked out on your bee butt. Humans share the same concerns, and consequently, they are constantly evaluating their place in the hierarchy of the tribe, the town, the gang, the organization. They judge their performance within any given hierarchy by posing the following three questions:

1. Am I good enough?
2. Am I performing my role well enough?
3. What does it take to maintain my place in the social hierarchy or to move up the ranks?

The need to fit in, to ascertain our status relative to what is needed to fit in, is a deeply wired one. A lot of our subconscious processing is about how we stack up. In today's world, our status is measured by how much money we have, by how cool we think we are, by how successful we are, by how much clout and power we have in our organization. That evaluation is so important to our self-perception relative to others. As a result, we are often our harshest critic, as the saying goes.

This critic within us is the subpersonality we call the **Standard Setter**.

What is key to evolutionary success across species is taking care of the young in such a way that more of them survive to adulthood and protecting all members of a group. Birds have nests, some mammals have protective herds or packs, and humans have families and homes and communities. Human beings ensure the functioning of the family and the community by investing in relationships; by being loving, nurturing, supportive, and caring toward others; by showing compassion. This is the subpersonality we call the **Relational**.

But a nestling can't stay in the nest forever. A child can't always just follow his or her parents. The drive that compels nestlings to leave the nest and become fledglings, and other animals' offspring to strike out on their own, is evident in humans, too. It's a drive that begins asserting itself during adolescence, which is why parents and their children often clash during this period. Kids want to break away from the nest, in one fashion or another, but often spend several years in turmoil about this. Sometimes they leave and come back. But at some point, most usually feel the need to take wing and fly away.

That need, that drive—and the courage to act on it—is the subpersonality we call **Autonomy**.

Here's another "built-in" conflict. Remember the more basic need for homeostasis, or stability? The drive for Autonomy is exactly the opposite: It's a need for change; for disruption; for upsetting the carefully arranged apple cart of the well-balanced family, in which the adults care for the children; for reorganizing the well-ordered community, in which members understand their respective roles.

And there's another conflict within our Inner Family. Not only do the drives for Autonomy and homeostasis inherently contradict each other, so do the drives for Autonomy and the Relational. This conflict boils down to either serving yourself (Autonomy) or serving others (the Relational).

These tensions are inherent, but they're not unresolvable. Consider marriage, which represents a compromise between two individuals. Individuals joined in matrimony have their own interests and drives, but each of them knows that in order to make the relationship work, they sometimes have to do things they may not want to do. So when a husband agrees to go and look at wallpaper for the new kitchen when there's a big football game on, he has probably resolved an inner conflict, bowing to the needs expressed by the Relational within him over the protests of Autonomy. Now, of course, not all husbands like football, and not all wives care about wallpaper, but neither would every couple resolve that conflict in the same way. Our genetic inheritance, combined with our experiences in life, makes the inner bargains with our subpersonalities a very individual thing. That's why some people are more compassionate toward others than most, and some people are more inclined to put their needs ahead of others'. That's also why some people never leave the small town they grew up in, while others bolt for the big city as soon as they can. There's no right or wrong here. We need people who are willing to make any of those choices between compassion and autonomy and stability, even if conflicts can arise among their often competing needs.

So if you're reading this and feeling that one of the subpersonalities in you is not strong enough, and that therefore you must somehow be flawed, think again. There really is no right or wrong. The needs, the subpersonalities, are in all of us, true, but they are not equally dominant. What is important, though, is that a balance is maintained; and that the less dominant needs are not completely silenced or squelched. All of them have a contribution to make.

But now let us continue to the next level in the hierarchy of needs. It's the need for organization. And we humans don't have a monopoly on it.

Think of beavers building dams and lodges. They cut down trees, figure out where to put the logs, stack and arrange them in just the right way. That's organization; that's getting things done! We humans build dams and lodges, too—and a lot more. We aren't just passive creatures who allow the environment around us to determine our fate. Very early on in our evolutionary history, we organized into packs of hunter-gatherers. Then we forged communities, and eventually, these gave rise to armies, governments, and corporations. This need for clarity in our own lives and in our interactions with others, this desire to create order out of chaos, is what we call the **Executive Manager**.

Potential conflict alert! Here comes the subpersonality that typically runs smack-dab into the Executive Manager. Here comes the problem solver, the one who likes to think outside the box. And that could mean the litter box. Yes, just as with organization, a strong suit of beavers, we humans don't have a monopoly on problem solving. When your cat figures out a clever way to climb up the furniture, the boxes, the lamps, and the walls in your living room in order to ascend to the top shelf of your bookcase, where it has spotted a cozy nook to snuggle up in, that feline is showing initiative. But, alas, beavers can't build the Golden Gate Bridge, and your cat will never compose a symphony or design a new app for your phone. They may be astute problem solvers, but they do not possess the human capacity for innovation—and not just in the arts, but in day-to-day living. This is the subpersonality we call the **Creative**.

The Executive Manager and the Creative are often in conflict. Just ask the people working in any advertising agency, any media corporation, any high-tech design firm, where both of these minds are at a premium. They represent two points at the opposite ends of the organization continuum. Creative minds tend to be disorganized minds. Creativity generally requires spontaneity, spontaneity means impulsivity, and impulsivity is the opposite of planning and a carefully thought-out approach.

Humans vary widely in terms of their Executive Manager and Creative quotients. In Coach Meg's work with her clients, this is one phenomenon she sees frequently. There is the talented innovator whose professional life is a mess because he or she forgets to return phone calls, doesn't arrive at meetings on time, and neglects to file expense reports. Then there is the fastidious, runs-like-clockwork manager who doesn't readily invent new ways of doing things and cannot respond and change quickly without first conducting a thorough analysis.

There's one last subpersonality that is exclusively human, and some might call it a curse. Unlike other species, humans have evolved to a point where they recognize that every life comes to an end. Such a brutal realization provides the impetus to find meaning, to seek a higher power or purpose, to believe in something greater than oneself. Of course, the making of meaning usually comes with more questions than answers, providing an inner conflict of its own. The subpersonality in charge of making meaning is what we call the **Meaning Maker**. While some may try to ignore it and others embrace it, it's a powerful member of the human Inner Family.

The Meaning Maker is sometimes in conflict with one of the subpersonalities, too. Recall that the Mindful Self is that state of mind in which one is able to observe, to be present, and to detach from one's needs. You could say that the Mindful Self is the ultimate expression of free will, as it's about you asserting as much control over a particular moment—your reactions, your thoughts, your needs—as you can manage. The Meaning Maker introduces the opposite perspective: it's about accepting and appreciating what is outside your control—for instance, your mortality, your destiny—and it takes a much longer view of life.

Hence, a conflict. *Another* conflict.

So you have nine discrete agendas to manage. And all these subpersonalities are rife with potential conflict. No wonder it's so hard to master oneself. It's like having a family with nine kids, each with their own needs and demands, all inside your head!

On any given day, several of your subpersonalities could be feeling good, and some could be suffering. Your mood at any given moment is the composite of all these subpersonalities.

You probably noticed that we presented these subpersonalities to you as a hierarchy, based on their appearance in an evolutionary timeline. But our experience is that while some of these subpersonalities may be more strident in one individual than another, the nine of them are more like a band of equals. You may not currently experience them in that way. The fact is, we need them all, despite their conflicting agendas.

The key to flourishing is not to eliminate these conflicts. As you have seen, they are innate. They're hardwired in our genes and reinforced by our experiences. No, the fact that you—or, to be specific, some part of you—is suffering or unhappy at any given moment is not unexpected. What we want to do is learn to manage and mediate those inner conflicts. That's how the competing inner voices, despite their different registers, can sing in harmony.

To return to the book *Divergent* and its dystopian society, the future, then, belongs not to those who know the single faction with which they are affiliated (the likes of selfless, peaceful, honest, brave, or knowledgeable), but to those who know who they are, those who recognize the multiple components that make up their personality. Let's continue on our quest to help you learn more about yours.

COACHING YOURSELF TO INNER HARMONY

We have devoted a great deal of space to exploring your emotions (the expressions of your subpersonalities) and their biological and evolutionary underpinnings. That's because we believe that the more you understand your emotions, the better you'll be able to handle the negative ones and harvest and amplify the positive ones. Understanding the nine subpersonalities will help you better understand the power and role of your particular set. You'll be better able to decode your emotional states. Once you have mastered that, you can consider the question "How can I better meet my needs?" That could lead you to make some big life decisions. Or not. For example, when you are involved in a serious relationship, you know you're going to lose some Autonomy, but your Relational capacity is going to make some gains. You will invariably ask how, and whether, your needs can be met.

On any given day, to what extent are all our needs being met? Few of us are meeting all our needs all the time. If you aren't making meaning, that can leave a hole. If you're not being adventurous, that can leave a hole. Understanding that can do more than tame the frenzy that results from the constant discord among the various subpersonalities. It can provide a road map to what you're able to do, and to what you need to do to have more equanimity.

So it's time to get better acquainted with your subpersonalities. Sure, you already know them; they are part of who you are, after all. But teasing out their individual voices in the ongoing internal dialogue, and the emotions that are expressing their needs or lack thereof, is something few of us are adept at doing.

What you need to do is what Coach Meg does with her clients: "I think you have an adult conversation with the parts of you that are thriving or suffering," she says. "It's basically a process of sitting down and interviewing yourself."

In the next few pages we will show you how Coach Meg used the self-interview to help one of her clients. This case dealt with a common conflict, one that we described in the previous section: the ongoing conflict in someone who is impulsive and innovative but disorganized. Or to put it in terms of our subpersonalities, someone who is having an ongoing inner debate between their Creative and Executive Manager capacities.

Remember, people who have a lot of creativity typically want to be spontaneous. They have little patience for rules or for doing things by the book. They'd prefer to tear up the book (hopefully not this one). They would rather have fun and play, even in their work life. That's not to say that they don't work hard or diligently, but they often view their work as a form of enjoyable play. They value freedom and impulsivity, like a horse that wants to run without a saddle and a bridle.

The Executive Manager represents the opposite of this. Those who are highly organized, whose Executive Manager is a powerful voice in their life, tend to be highly structured and organized. They don't go out to play, at least not in their workplace. They seek clarity and precision and engage in careful decision making. They thrive on the structure and discipline of the saddle and bridle. When the Creative is dominant, the Executive Manager is often ignored or sublimated. And don't forget the other seven subpersonalities, which also impact the overall weather forecast.

This is a situation that is fairly typical. A creative entrepreneur—a writer or a graphic designer or a filmmaker—is having problems because his or her need for impulsivity and drive for freedom has led to an abdication of responsibilities. Being so "free" and creative, has also made this individual sloppy and disorganized to the point that his or her work and personal lives are suffering.

Often, such individuals come to Coach Meg for help.

Which brings us to Pete, one of the clients who benefited from Coach Meg's use of the self-interview. Pete, who was in his midthirties, was a design director at an advertising agency.

He was very creative—his work had won a number of industry awards—and very disorganized. So much so that it was affecting his job and his marriage. The final straw was when Pete pulled a Don Draper–like disappearing act at a big client meeting one afternoon. He had spaced it out completely and had gone off to scout locations for an upcoming photo shoot on another project, and he was hastily summoned back to the office by a frantic and angry call from his boss in the conference room. It was then decided that he needed to get a handle on this issue.

Pete met with Meg, who, after listening to his story, explained to him about the subpersonalities. "Once he understood the distinct personality parts, I told him that now we were going to hold a meeting that all of them needed to attend," she says. "This was one meeting he couldn't be late for, because it was basically a meeting of everything that was going on in his head." Since all of Pete's nine subpersonalities were contributing to his inner dialogue, all of them were invited to speak in this session, which we refer to as a Roll Call.

This kind of session isn't voodoo, a séance, or an exorcism, in which spirits from the beyond are summoned or confronted. This is simply a matter of identifying a voice that's already contributing to the inner dialogue, something that is ongoing in all of us, and then asking that voice essentially to speak up and say what it needs to say.

"We imagine it as a round table meeting with yourself," Coach Meg told Pete. "Like when the boss holds a staff meeting to discuss improved performance and asks each department to provide an update of what's going one and how they can help. That's what we're doing here. Trying to get a sense from each subpersonality, each of your needs, as to how this issue is impacting them and what can be done about it."

The issue here was Pete's unbridled, free-rein creativity, which had led to missed appointments, snafus, unreturned e-mails, and other problems of disorganization. Meg asks her clients to try to tune in to all parts of their personality and to report what they're saying. In Pete's case, the feedback sounded something like this:

Autonomy: "We're not going to accomplish our goals and move forward in life if we continue to be so sloppy and disorganized. We need to get better organized."

The Body Regulator: "This disorder is so stressful. It's not healthy! I'm losing sleep. I'm not eating well. We need to fix this."

Confidence: "I've been read the riot act by my boss and my wife for messing up on so many deadlines and appointments. That's hurting my confidence. I don't feel we can get things done without figuring out a way to get more structured."

The Curious Adventurer: "I don't like the idea of getting more structured. It doesn't sound like much of an adventure. But you know, if we got better organized and could meet our deadlines, maybe you wouldn't have to go in to work on Saturdays, and we'd be able to go rock climbing, which we've wanted to do for years."

The Executive Manager: "I'm tired of being shouted down. Let me out of the basement. The Creative takes over all the time. I'm not getting the opportunity to do what I do well."

The Relational: "You're messing up your relationships, because you're unreliable. Your wife is ticked off, and your friends are annoyed. And think about how you've inconvenienced them every time you forgot you were supposed to pick up the kids from soccer or you canceled a lunch date at the last minute with your buddy!"

The Standard Setter: "If we're going to achieve more, you need to get more organized. You're talented, but you're not accomplishing enough."

The Meaning Maker: "You know you have talent and were meant to do what you do. But you might be able to do it better if you just got a little better organized."

Now it was the Creative against the other eight voices. While that was undoubtedly one of the dominant voices in Pete's personality, it was now outnumbered and had to relent. Coach Meg encouraged Pete to listen to his Executive Manager.

How, you might wonder, did Pete end up addressing the issue of his disorganization once he held his inner meeting, his Roll Call? "He had the ability to come up with a solution," Coach Meg says. "But as that voice was telling him, he had to learn to stop ignoring what it was saying." The solution was simply that Pete began to spend not days or hours, but minutes—specifically, ten minutes every three to four hours—attending to the organizational aspects of his life or job.

So instead of taking a coffee break from the fun part of his job, he now takes a "structure break." He reviews his e-mail and responds, goes over his calendar, returns any calls. Basically, he just learned to stay on top of things. Clockwork efficiency and rigid organization are never going to be Pete's strong suits, but that wasn't the point. "His Creative continues to be a dominant voice, a dominant drive and need in his life," Meg says. "The difference is that now it's not the only voice he listens to."

IDENTIFY YOURSELF!

One of the longest-running and most successful game shows in American television history is *To Tell the Truth*, in which four celebrity panelists (Kitty Carlisle, Tom Poston, Peggy Cass, and Orson Bean were among the regulars in the 1960s) attempted to identify a contestant with an unusual, even newsworthy occupation or experience. Over the decades many of the contestants were important, even famous personalities at the time they appeared on the show. They just weren't recognizable faces.

Each contestant was accompanied by two impostors who sat alongside deftly answering the questions fired at them by the panel. The challenge for the panelists was to determine which of the three individuals was the genuine person behind the story. The big reveal involved the host of the program asking the person to identify him- or herself to the panel and the audience. This request was always delivered in the form of a memorable line, "Will the *real* [name] please stand up?" So when, for example, Rosa Parks was asked at the end of her segment to identify herself, the host intoned, "Will the *real* Rosa Parks please stand up?" Hunter Thompson, Alex Haley, Orville Redenbacher, Berry Gordy, and Tony LaRussa—all of whom appeared as contestants on the show—were asked their version of this question at the end of their segments, as were all the other contestants. "Will the *real* . . . please stand up?" would become a catchphrase (one used by rapper Eminem in song lyrics).

Just as, say, Berry Gordy, founder of the Motown record label, might not be easy to pick out in a crowd, it's not always easy to discern the voices of your Executive Manager or your Confidence, even though you may know and feel their effects every day. Remember this when you first try to distinguish the various voices that make up your inner dialogue and drive so much of your behavior. In your state of mindfulness, you should feel free to ask—silently to yourself, or even out loud, if you feel comfortable doing so—that same question from *To Tell the Truth*.

"Will the *real* Executive Manager please stand up? Will the *real* part of me that is concerned with taking control, please stand up now and make yourself known?"

"Will my Autonomy capacity please stand up? Can I hear that voice?"

These voices are already present; they're chattering away all the time. We're trying to organize them, trying to figure out who's saying what, and why. As you have read, there are at least nine that are common to most people, and there may be a few that are unique to you. You may not hear any the first time you tune in, at least not clearly. "Sometimes clients ask, 'What will these voices sound like?'" Coach Meg says. "I think they're expecting them to have an English accent or a higher register, or to sound like they're coming from someone else's mouth." It's not quite that dramatic. Remember that you're already listening to them every waking hour. They will sound like you, because they *are* you. Or aspects of you.

It's likely that a few will come in loud and clear. These are the dominant aspects of your personality—the "loudest" members of your Inner Family, so to speak—reflecting your greatest needs and strengths. When you start to tune in, initially, you may only be able to name and recognize these loudest ones. The others may not "speak up" at first, because they may not be used to asserting themselves. But while they may not be available to you right away, they do have something to say. These listening moments are opportunities for you to become better balanced and more aware of your unmet needs, and while it will take time and a little patience and practice, you will eventually get the messages.

Here's an example of this: Fitness professionals love to talk about "listening to your body." Well, whether the personal trainer at the local gym is aware of this or not, you now know that he or she is referring to the part of your personality we call the Body Regulator. If you're not eating right or exercising, and if you're stressed out and not sleeping well, then clearly, this part of you is not getting your attention. It's a voice that's being drowned out by other needs, which happen to be stronger right now. But whether it's a dominant voice or a meeker one, every voice has a perspective you need to hear—which is why it's wise to listen, as opposed to going through life without ever making sense of the dialogue within.

What you will find over time is that some parts of your personality are feeling fulfilled and other parts are not. The energy that enables you to go forth and accomplish great things in life comes from those parts that are doing well. But if you have parts that are not doing well, then *you* are not doing well. When you're utilizing your inner capacities fully, you're going to be happier, healthier, and more successful.

The most dominant voices of your personality will make themselves plain. The others, as we said, will take time to tease out. Which aspects of your personality are which? What will they say? And perhaps more importantly, what will you do with the information? These are the questions that we will address in the upcoming chapters, as we take a close-up look at each of the nine major subpersonalities.

3

MEET YOUR EMOTIONS

Emotions get a bad rap in literature, in song, even on the Internet.

"The advantage of the emotions is that they lead us astray," writes Oscar Wilde in his 1891 classic *The Picture of Dorian Gray*.

In "Emotional Rescue," on their 1980 album by the same name, the Rolling Stones sing about coming "to your emotional rescue," as if one must be saved from one's feelings.

On an Internet forum, a young woman asks the question "Why am I so emotional?" Respondents rush to offer suggestions to combat this affliction, as if she were discussing halitosis or cellulitis.

We'd like to suggest a different view of human emotions, one that doesn't consider them inherently bad or harmful; that doesn't insist that they must be controlled or mastered; that doesn't believe you should be ashamed of them or, at the other extreme, prouder of them than you are of your ability to see or hear. We should be *grateful* for our five senses, which guide us through the world, and we should be just as grateful for our emotions. Because *they* can guide us as surely as our eyes and ears, if we know how to use them.

"Emotions organize—rather than disrupt—rational thinking," write Dacher Keltner and Paul Ekman in a July 2015 *New York Times* op-ed piece entitled "The Science of 'Inside Out.'" "Traditionally, in the history of Western thought, the prevailing view has been that emotions are enemies of rationality and disruptive of cooperative social relations." Keltner and Ekman, two University of California psychologists who served as the scientific consultants to the 2015 Pixar film *Inside Out*, go on to point out that the real purpose of our emotions is to "guide our perceptions of the world, our memories of the past and even our moral judgments of right and wrong, most typically in ways that enable effective responses to the current situation."

Katherine T. Peil of Northeastern University views the emotions as something even more fundamental, like another sense, or as she puts it, "an entire sensory system . . . that guides biological self-regulation." In her 2014 paper entitled "Emotion: The Self-Regulatory Sense," published in *Global Advances in Health and Medicine,* she recasts emotions not as some sort of human affliction or weakness, nor as an inconvenient aspect of our psyches that sometimes makes us say or do foolish and regrettable things, but rather as a sensory system, like sight, hearing, and touch, that provides us with an ongoing stream of what she terms "self-relevant" information.

The purpose of this emotional system, she argues, is self-regulatory, meaning that it helps to control or direct our behavior. That direction is based on our needs. Essentially, Peil maintains that our emotions are telling us what those needs are. Our genes drive our needs, which, in turn, talk to us through our emotions.

Such needs might seem obvious. Basic needs, such as food,

shelter, and so forth, are common to all of us. Others, which vary in their degree of importance or triviality, we proclaim on a daily basis: "I need a new car," "I need a vacation," and "I need a better system for organizing my recipes."

Our advice on the vacation: Bermuda is nice this time of year. Seriously, you probably don't need the help of a book for those kinds of needs. What we want you to understand is that sometimes your needs arise from deeper, less-visited places within you, and that these places must be explored, their messages interpreted and understood before you can act on them. It's often these underlying needs that are the root cause of many other concerns in our life or the reason we are dissatisfied, even if we don't really know why.

Let's take a sublime human quality such as creativity. A cluster of genes likely underpins your particular style of creativity. Perhaps you inherited your mother's musical talent, your grandfather's writing ability, maybe someone else's creative way of looking at situations in a "noncreative" field (outside of accounting, we hasten to add, for any IRS professionals reading this). All of them contributed to your creativity.

This cluster of genes is basically a strength, a drive, and a need—and it needs to be used. These genes don't want to be dormant or suppressed; they want to do their work! So let's say you've got this combination of "creative" genes, and you live or work in an environment that's based on routine and structure, where there is little room for creativity. This creative need of yours is not likely to be met in such an environment. How is that going to make you feel? Probably unhappy and dissatisfied.

There you go. Your emotions are communicating to you a need that's being felt at the deepest level of your makeup.

As for those bundles of "creative" genes you inherited from

Mom and Granddad and others, they express themselves as one of the nine subpersonalities we've discussed in the previous chapters, through the language of emotions. Your emotional "sense" in the previous example could simply be saying to you, "We've got to get into a different environment, find activities where we can be more creative." Often, though the message may not be as direct or as easily understood. As creativity often is closely linked with impulsivity, it may mean that because your creativity is being thwarted in your work life, your needs will act it out in some way, and maybe not a positive one. For instance, you might act impulsively when it comes to eating, online shopping, or talking.

This is where Katherine Peil's theory on the sensory, self-regulatory role of emotions links with the concept of the subpersonalities, which we examined in detail in the last chapter. The Creative, you may recall, is one of those nine subpersonalities. These are powerful drives, and if they're thwarted, the negative emotions that arise will let us know.

Here's another example of how the emotions are often conduits for the subpersonalities to articulate their needs. Coach Meg had a client named Amy, who worked in health care. A big part of Amy's life force came from a desire for autonomy. By making an inventory of Amy's subpersonalities—something we will show you how to do later in this book—Coach Meg actually determined that Amy's Autonomy, Creative, and Curious Adventurer were the powerful drivers in her psyche. Yet Amy wasn't using any of them. In particular, her Autonomy had been suppressed for years. "She was in a job where none of the qualities associated with Autonomy were really valued or encouraged," says Coach Meg. "You could hear it in her voice. Her energy was restrained. The Executive Manager, by necessity, was running the show and was not letting these life forces, these dominant capacities express themselves."

This is another important point, and one that most of us likely know from experience. Sometimes the messages we receive from our emotions are conflicted, even contradictory. That's not because our self-regulatory sense is out of whack. It's more likely a reflection of the lack of congruence, for many of us, between our inner drives and capacities and the reality of our lives. Not everyone—few of us, in truth—are in job situations where we are doing exactly what we feel we should be doing, where our talents or abilities are utilized to the fullest extent. There may be very sound reasons why that is so, but practical reality will not mute the inherent drives of your genes—expressed through your subpersonalities—to do what they're designed to do. It's not that they're impractical; they're just programmed that way!

Decoding those conflicting voices and emotions helps us tame the frenzy in our minds and start the process toward developing a more fulfilled and happier life.

Back to Amy, Coach Meg's client in health care. One reason she remained in a job where she was closely supervised and had little autonomy was that she was well compensated and she enjoyed a good deal of job security. These were important considerations given that she had to earn an income that was sufficient to raise two young children. Still, Amy was depressed and frustrated. Even though on one level she knew that the rational choice was to stay in her current job, her drive for autonomy was so strong that her lack of it in the workplace was expressed through negative emotions that sometimes seemed to overwhelm her.

Coach Meg did not suggest to Amy that in order to meet the

increasingly loud demands of her Autonomy, she must quit her job and become self-employed, which was certain to afford her all the autonomy she wanted, but none of the regular, predictable income she needed. Maybe she could do that when the kids were no longer as dependent on her. Instead, Coach Meg suggested ways in which Amy could allow her autonomous inclinations to do their thing. Or, as Peil would say, allow these emotions—which she refers to in "Emotion: The Self-Regulatory Sense" as "nothing less than a biological value system, informing us of universally right and wrong states of balanced being and becoming"—to do just that, to balance and regulate. In Amy's case, it would involve transforming her job in a way that allowed her more autonomy or trying to find a new job, one where she would have more independence and autonomy.

Since finding a new job was not an easy task, Amy followed Coach Meg's advice about her present job, proposing to her supervisor some changes in her job description that would give her a little more autonomy. Her boss agreed, and now, even if Amy's powerful driving force of Autonomy is not guiding her work life, at least it's no longer completely muted. Since it is now playing a larger role in her work, she is no longer quite as anxious or dissatisfied with her life.

When we view the emotions as a system of self-regulation, the way Katherine Peil has so brilliantly theorized, we can see them in a different light. We can view them not as a burden, not as an inconvenience, not as something that we are saddled with and that always seem to rear their head at the wrong time. No, we can now see emotions, particularly negative emotions, the way they should be seen: as messengers.

Social psychologist Barbara Fredrickson of the University of

North Carolina–Chapel Hill has studied the biology and impact of positive emotions. Her research suggests that an optimal mix of emotions is required for our brain to function well and for us to maintain good physical health. While the ideal ratio of positive to negative emotions is a matter of debate, it's generally believed that you need both, but with a good surplus of the positive.

Positive emotions broaden our horizons, help us see the big picture, and allow us to be more flexible and adaptable to fluid situations. They enable us to focus better, they help us tame the frenzy, and they help us with strategic thinking. They also may help us on a more basic physiological level. Research conducted by Fredrickson and her colleagues has shown that positive emotions are associated with improved nervous and cardiovascular system function, improved mental well-being, and even longevity.

Fredrickson has moved the research on positive emotions forward by constructing what she calls the broaden-and-build theory of positive emotions. According to this theory, positive emotions beget more positive emotions, resulting in a reservoir of such emotions, which are available when needed. She and her colleagues Michele Tugade and Lisa Feldman Barrett elaborate on this idea in an article entitled "Psychological Resilience and Positive Emotional Granularity: Examining the Benefits of Positive Emotions on Coping and Health," published in the *Journal of Personality* in 2004.

> *According to the broaden-and-build theory, positive emotions can momentarily broaden one's scopes of thought and allow for flexible attention, which, in turn, can improve one's well-being. Over time, and with repeated experiences of positive*

emotions, this broadened mind-set might become habitual. By consequence, then, the often-incidental effect of experiencing a positive emotion is an increase in one's personal resources. Importantly, the arsenal of personal resources produced by positive emotions can be drawn on in times of need and used to plan for future outcomes, which may be valuable in facilitating healthy behavioral practices.

While positive emotions can indeed be a powerful force now and in the future, negative emotions are also important to our mental health and well-being. If we follow Peil's hypothesis that the emotions are another one of our senses, then attempting to block out negative emotions would be akin to closing our eyes at the sight of anything unpleasant. Naturally, you might want to do that, but as we all know, sometimes we must face things as they are and not live in denial. Same with negative emotions. They're basically signaling that we need something, whether it's a new adventure in life or a new approach to our nutrition.

Here is something else you should know about your emotions. The positive ones, though so important for health, tend to be fleeting. The negative ones are stickier; they stay with you, stick in your craw. So part of our challenge in developing our emotional intelligence is to create more positive emotions—or at least learn how to savor the ones we have—and to share them with others. (Fredrickson's research shows that sharing your positivity—feeling good *and* making others feel good—is one way in which positive emotions can improve physical health.)

One more positive thing about positive emotions: they make it easier to cope with those nasty negative emotions that linger. Such emotions can be draining, depleting; some can even be physically painful. But as painful and distressing as they can be, negative emotions are often the ones that lead us to breakthroughs and to revelations about ourselves that are life changing.

Notice that we don't say that we can banish negative emotions forever. Of course we can't. This book is about helping you create a positive inner culture—and in the process, taming your frenzy and putting yourself on the road to a happier, more productive, and satisfying life. It is not about eliminating negative emotions. You never will. They're like clouds. They'll keep coming back. Some days will be brilliantly sunny and clear. On other days there may be cloud cover. For good reason. There are always needs that are unmet; there are always changing needs—all expressed through emotions. Some of them are situational (you're stuck in traffic); some of them are deeper seated.

The real question is, exactly what messages are these emotions, both positive and negative, delivering? What are the needs, unmet or met, that lay deep in the recesses of our mind, our heart, our DNA? If only it were as easy as meeting the needs for food, water, and shelter, as easy as opening the refrigerator or a bottle of water or turning up the heat on a cold day! Or, in the case of the traffic jam, finding an alternate route. There is little ambiguity about those needs, the basic ones for food, water, and shelter, and the one for a less stressful commute home from work. In those cases, the message is crystal clear and urgent. But when we are dealing with the complexities and variables of human behavior, the higher-level aspects of our psyche, it's not.

However, we can learn to *identify* those emotions—a key step to decoding these inner needs and, in turn, shedding light on the "inner you," that complex interplay of your subpersonalities and your interior dialogue.

In the next section, we will show you how.

THE SIX STEPS OF EMOTIONAL DECODING

It's time to take a look at your emotional weather forecast. And you can do that in six steps. This exercise is not necessarily going to provide you with answers as to what is ailing you. But by recognizing the question that's being asked or, more precisely, the emotion that's making itself felt, this should put you in a better place.

You can "forecast" anywhere and anytime. It requires that you first try to get into that state of mindfulness we discussed earlier. So sit down, relax, and try to put yourself in the moment. Ask yourself, "How am I feeling?" The answer will lead you to Step 1:

Step 1: Noticing and naming the emotion
Okay, so how *are* you feeling? Notice the emotion present in your answer to that question and *name* it. "I am feeling angry." "I am feeling anxious." "I am feeling calm." Try to gauge the intensity of those feelings. Are you feeling *really* anxious, or do you just have a vague sense of unease, a sense of disquiet? Try to identify the emotion and describe it in as much detail as possible, and do this nonjudgmentally and objectively, as you would approach everything when in a state of mindfulness.

Step 2: Acceptance
You've identified and labeled the emotion. Now relax, breathe, and accept it. Don't question why you're feeling this way; don't reject the emotion. Don't judge it. This is what you are feeling. Don't beat yourself up over it. No "I wish I didn't panic. I wish I wasn't stressed. I wish I didn't feel this way." Remember, this emotion is

a messenger, and you don't want to kill the messenger! Besides, pushing back against a negative emotion will result in more negative emotions or even adverse physiological responses. Your stomach can get in a knot, you might start sweating, and you could even get physically sick over it. Don't! Don't try to push back against these emotions. Accept that they are here, that they are trying to communicate something to you, and understand that you are about to take steps to act on that information.

Step 3: Appreciation

Remember Peil's theory that emotions can be viewed as another sense, like seeing and hearing and touching? Aren't we grateful for our eyes and ears and fingers? We should be. And similarly, we should be grateful for having this emotional system that is really designed to help us feel better. Take a moment to appreciate the emotion. It's helping you, it's guiding you, it's pushing you, and it's telling you what you need. Be glad your brain is sending you this message. This appreciation will help you to accept the emotion, and it will also help put you in the proper frame of mind to deal with it in a more dispassionate, effective manner, as opposed to letting it overwhelm you.

Step 4: Connection

"Smile and the world smiles with you. Cry and you cry alone." It's a nice little proverb—and like any good proverb, there's some truth to it, in terms of the value of sharing positive emotions, the way Barbara Fredrickson suggests. But in actuality, when you cry, you are not crying alone. You are not unhappy alone. Everyone has negative emotions, some worse than others, yes, but there is not a human being alive who has never felt even a passing twang of remorse, guilt, anxiety . . . you name it. In fact, you *have* named it (in step 1). Whatever that emotion you are now feeling, remember that you are not alone in feeling that way.

Dr. Kristin Neff of the University of Texas at Austin cites "connection" as one of the three components of self-compassion. The other two are mindfulness and self-kindness. We've talked about the former in this book, and the latter is always a good idea. But being kind and compassionate to yourself and others doesn't just mean that we all hold hands around the campfire and sing "Kumbaya" because we're all unhappy about something together. It's a reminder that you are not an isolated black hole of despair in a universe filled with twinkling stars. Everyone has these emotions; it's a function of being human. Many people have worked through them in order to find understanding and achieve happier, more fulfilled lives. You can, too.

Step 5: Compassion

For all their sophistication—expressing, as they sometimes do, some of the most complex higher-level human needs—negative emotions are like crying babies. They want your attention, they want a hug, they want to be safe and not alone, and they want to know you care. So simply crossing your hands over your heart or giving yourself a little mental hug, a pat on the back, or a high five can help. It may sound silly, but some would argue that this ability to feel compassion over your own suffering or unhappiness is the most important step in this process. At a 2013 Harvard Medical School conference, Thich Nhat Hanh said that "mindful compassion teaches you how to suffer well." For our purposes, let's put the emphasis on the *well*. Having a little heart toward your own heart softens the sting of these negative emotions.

Step 6: Curiosity
Now we can start to probe the meaning of this emotion. "I wonder why I'm feeling this way? Is there something I could be doing differently?" We are beginning the process of tuning in to that Inner Family, of connecting our emotions to our nine subpersonalities. You can begin to think about what need isn't being addressed and why. Again, this is a nonjudgmental analysis. No beating yourself up over what you think may have caused you to feel this way. Or, just as bad, blaming others. This is a step in which we go, "Hmmm."

Okay, you're done! Now, go back to what you were doing—except, hopefully, you are feeling a little better, a little calmer now. You don't necessarily have to solve the issue right now. You want to settle things sufficiently, so that you don't feel frenzied and paralyzed by these emotions. Following these six steps will do just that, and that process will help set the stage for more productive thinking as we probe deeper into the underlying causes of your concerns (that "hmmm" part of step 6 is, in a way, the initial step in that process).

Here's an example of how the six steps of decoding the emotion can help defuse a bad situation and help turn it around. Let's say you just had an argument with your child. You are upset with yourself because you weren't a good listener. You were impulsive, you said some things you shouldn't have, and now you're angry at yourself—as angry as you were with your child a few minutes ago.

First, name the emotion: "I'm too angry, and I overreacted. And I wish I had not done that."

Then acceptance and appreciation: "I didn't behave well, and now I'm annoyed. Not denying it. That's what it is. The best I could muster in that moment. I'm not going to make excuses. I'm just going to sit with the truth of it and then ponder objectively how I could have done better. I know I'm angry at myself, and it's justified. And I'm going to try to use this experience to learn, so that I do not react the same way next time."

Now connect: "I'm not the only person I know that's a bad listener!"

Next, self-compassion: "It feels bad to be angry at myself. I just really want a good relationship with my child, and instead, I fight with her, and now I'm down on myself. This is a sucky feeling."

Curiosity: "What could I do better next time? She's still discovering who she is and testing her boundaries, but I realize she's still trying to do her best. I'm going to talk to her and apologize for overreacting. And I'm going to think about how I can better handle this kind of situation next time."

As we forge ahead, let's first make sure we've connected some dots. In chapter 1, we talked about the importance of mindfulness, which, as we just showed, is the way we can more calmly and objectively look at our emotions. The emotions are tied to our so-called Inner Family, those subpersonalities we outlined in the Introduction and also delineated further in chapters 1 and 2. Which of these nine members of your Inner Family is this negative emotion linked to? Which of these nine entities of the psyche is trying to tell you something through the vehicle (or the self-regulatory sense) of this emotion? If you're unhappy or unfulfilled, we need to find the part of you that is unhappy or unfulfilled. Is it Autonomy, your Creative, your Meaning Maker, or your Curious Adventurer? If you're lacking confidence, we need to find the part of you that doubts yourself. Is it your Executive Manager, your Standard Setter, your Relational capacity? Now you're starting to understand your inner frenzy, because you recognize what you need to do to help tame it. Because emotional states can be complex, we'll show you how to deal with each in the upcoming chapters.

Finally, remember the power of emotions. We've talked about them as another sensory system. Consider this observation from a woman whose conventional sensory system was compromised, and who learned to read and experience the world, in large part, through her emotions. "The best and most beautiful things in the world cannot be seen or even touched, but just felt in the heart," wrote Helen Keller in an 1891 letter.

DR. EDDIE:
A Case Study in the Healing Power of Emotions

In a 2013 article entitled "Is Pain a Construct of the Mind?" in the magazine *Scientific American Mind*, neuroscientist and science writer Stephen L. Macknik makes the interesting observation, based on a number of recent studies, that pain is more than a physiological response. It's an emotion, as well.

If that's so, my patients are highly emotional. Because they come to me in pain, often in extreme pain. As a specialist in physical medicine and rehabilitation, I treat their sore knees, aching backs, and stiff necks. I observe them walking into the exam room slowly and tentatively, if they walk at all. They wince as the unconscious, well-practiced movement of reaching over-head or putting on a jacket causes lancinating agony due to an inflamed shoulder. A simple sneeze ignites a pinched nerve in the lower back, causing an audible gasp.

The physical pain from their ailments is not the only source of my patients' suffering. They suffer when the physical pain leads to an array of emotions, which they carry as a burden. They are angered by their body's betrayal and fearful of worsening aches and declining function. They are fatigued and irritable when throbbing disrupts their sleep, and frustrated when nothing seems to alleviate their discomfort. Even those who are normally even tempered and well mannered or have a sunny disposition are cranky and short when they are in pain. They grieve over an inability to play sports, walk their dogs, or even sit comfortably and watch a movie. Confidence evaporates as treatments fail and physicians shake their heads. Although I am trained to treat my patients' pain, it is only by addressing their suffering and the associated emotions that relief is available to those with chronic pain. I work with patients to call on their Inner Family in an at-tempt to regain control of their lives.

During a recent visit, one of my patients, Katherine, a fifty-two-year-old college professor with debilitating chronic back pain, described her experience. "At my worst, I am in despair and not sure how I can make it through the next several hours,

let alone forever." In a sense her Body Regulator was screaming so loudly in anguish that no other voice could be heard. She
had to rally herself just to show up for our next appointment. I
entered the exam room, where Katherine sat stock-still, as if set
in concrete.

"It hurts when I move," she explained.

I paused for a moment to shake her hand and look her in
the eye.

Her mouth creaked a perfunctory "How are you?"

Running behind schedule, I answered, "Late . . . but what else
is new?" Just this mild attempt at humor in the darkness of her
dejection melted the ice a bit. A sliver of a smile creased her
face, and her intensity softened. Her unnatural stillness eased
as her mind began to open and perhaps become a bit more creative. I asked her how I could help.

"If you could cure me, it would be best," she replied. "But just
listening to me is a good start."

We had long ago exhausted the simple fixes for her pain that
I could administer to her. She needed to regain some Autonomy
and Confidence to reduce her suffering and her sense that the
pain had pushed her life off the tracks.

When I inquired about her mood and her emotions, she quietly
confided in me her growing sense that nothing would ever help
her. She did, however, become more animated as she expressed
her anger over and frustration with the physical therapist's enthu-
siastic and energetic attempts to try yet another new treatment.
"In a way, it felt better to be angry with her than to feel the numb-
ness of despair that I will never get better," she confessed.

I attempted to access Katherine's Creative and her Curious
Adventurer to improve her open-mindedness and idea generation as we began to explore further modifications or options to

relieve pain and improve function. "We've tried different treatments to reduce your pain and get you more active. What was the best part of the physical therapy?"

She thought about it. "Well, now that you ask, going on the stationary bike at least got my body moving. Pedaling away on a bicycle made me feel a bit like my old self."

This realization sounded like a break in the clouds of her gloom. I attempted to bolster her autonomy and self-reliance by asking her how she would like to proceed.

"Well, my neighbor has a bicycle she doesn't use and is willing to lend me. I suppose I could try that at home."

Indeed, despite Katherine's severe pain, she began to ride the stationary bike slowly but regularly at home. At a subsequent appointment she reported that while her pain had not improved, she was able to do more for herself and was therefore feeling a bit better. I endeavored to engage more of her Inner Family when she acknowledged the improvement in her Autonomy now that she could sit comfortably a bit longer and could go for a walk outside, thanks to her improved endurance from her bicycling.

"What would it take to get you back to teaching at least one class next semester?"

She smiled as her mind drifted back to the campus and the classrooms where she had spent so much of her working life. "I'm not sure I can make the drive three times per week to campus, but I would really love to be engaged again with students. It would get me out of my own head." She nodded firmly—was this the voice of Confidence asserting itself?—and then looked me in the eye. "Getting back in front of the classroom is what I want."

She was yearning for the social connection with students but lacked the confidence that her body was ready for the challenge. She accessed her Creative and settled on the interim steps of overseeing an online course from home and driving to the campus once or twice a week to go to the library.

Her chronic back pain had continued, but she was now regaining contact with the rest of her Inner Family, enabling her to reconnect with her love of teaching and acknowledge her need to first improve her autonomy and self-reliance. Her Creative voice was providing options to her now that she could stop and listen, and her Confidence was willing to give these suggestions a try. I suspect she'll be inspiring a class full of undergraduates again in the near future—and feeling much better for it.

This patient isn't cured, not by a long shot. She may never be. But what she has done, I think, is instructive, and it is consistent with what Coach Meg would advise all her clients:

* Work to overcome the shouting of one inner voice (as my patient did with her Body Regulator) so that you can access the other voices. It is in the full chorus of the Inner Family that the secrets lie to taming your frenzy and better organizing your emotions.
* Remain open to the full palate of your emotions. The inner voices express these emotions. Even negative emotions, such as fear and anger, can energize and prompt action.
* Just a touch of humor can improve open-mindedness and curiosity.
* Don't be afraid to set a big goal (e.g., my patient returning to teaching), while still taking the smaller steps (riding the stationary bicycle).
* Taking small steps can provide a glimmer of hope and improve self-efficacy.

4

AUTONOMY

For more than three decades, University of Rochester psychologists Edward Deci and Richard Ryan have delved deep into the question of human motivation: Are we driven by external factors—grades, annual job evaluations, rating systems, the opinions of others? Or does our motivation come from within—from our own interests, curiosity, or values?

Most likely, they have concluded, it's both; and in the process, they have created an influential meta-theory on the driving forces that underlie human behavior. "The interplay between the extrinsic forces acting on persons and the intrinsic motives and needs inherent in human nature," they write on their Web site, Self-DeterminationTheory.org, "is the territory of Self-Determination Theory."

Just like some of the theories of other influential thinkers we have discussed in earlier chapters, Deci and Ryan's self-determination theory (SDT) is one of the cornerstones of this book and our approach to helping you organize your emotions, tame the frenzy, and thrive.

The central principle of SDT is that there are three basic psychological needs essential to healthy social and cognitive development and functioning:

Competence, or what we call Confidence in this book.
Relatedness, or what we call the Relational.
Autonomy, a biggie when it comes to flourishing.

"To the extent that the needs are ongoingly satisfied," Deci and Ryan write on their Web site, "people will develop and function effectively and experience wellness, but to the extent that they are thwarted, people more likely evidence ill-being and nonoptimal functioning."

Clearly, autonomy is important. But what does it really mean? *Merriam-Webster's Collegiate Dictionary,* eleventh edition, defines *autonomy* as "the quality or state of being self-governing; especially: the right of self-government." In a 2000 journal article, "The 'What' and the 'Why' of Goal Pursuits: Human Needs and the Self-Determination of Behavior," Deci and Ryan write that autonomy "refers to volition—the organismic desire to self-organize experience and behavior and to have activity be concordant with one's integrated sense of self."

Autonomy finds its expression in popular culture. There are countless examples of this. For instance, in the late 1960s, singer Sammy Davis Jr. had a hit song that could be called the national anthem of Autonomy. "I've gotta be me," Sammy declared in the song's surging chorus. "I've gotta be me." Maybe it's no surprise that "I've Gotta Be Me" was a hit, reaching number eleven on the

Billboard Hot 100 chart in 1969. It spoke powerfully to something inside all of us.

AUTONOMY IN THE FAMILY

Of the nine subpersonalities in our Inner Family, which provide the inner dialogue that drives our behavior, we believe that Autonomy may be numero uno.

We want to self-determine, we want to self-actualize, and we want to find ourselves. We want to find our own drumbeat. We want to be authentic.

The autonomous drive is the one that motivates adolescents to leave home to attend college, join the military, volunteer in Africa, or bum around Europe for a summer.

The autonomous drive is the one that compels middle-aged adults working in large organizations to question their career choices, to chafe under the strictures of a hierarchy or a bureaucracy, to dream about starting their own business.

The need for autonomy drives revolutions, as well as revelations. We wake up one morning and finally decide we've had enough of whatever it is.

The drive for autonomy has changed the course of history. It is what led a group of fractious American colonists to declare their independence from what they saw as an oppressive, controlling mother country in 1776. It is what compelled many to leave the nations of Europe and other countries for the promise of a better life in America—a life in which they could, at least in theory, be judged as individuals on their merits, not according to their parents' or family's status. It is what inspired a college dropout named

Steve Jobs and his friend Steve Wozniak to thumb their noses at established corporations and invent a new computer—and, it could be argued, a new society—in the garage of Jobs's childhood home.

As those examples suggest, autonomy seems to be a particularly powerful drive in American society. Indeed, there are some who would argue that in an increasingly interdependent world, we may even have too much autonomy.

We'll leave that controversy to the cultural theorists and macroeconomists. Coach Meg says it's a top issue with her clients. "What we're always aiming for . . . in our practice and in this book . . . is to get people flourishing," she says. "That means finding the unmet needs. What are they? A key one is often autonomy."

A FAMILY SIT-DOWN: FOUR QUESTIONS FOR NINE SUBPERSONALITIES

With Autonomy, as with each of the other eight members of your Inner Family, it's useful to ask a series of questions. Some of these questions you can probably answer right off the bat. Others will require that you get into that state of mindfulness we discussed in depth in chapter 1 and "call out" this part of yourself, this subpersonality, that is, focus in on the part that strives for authenticity, for autonomy.

Engaging in this form of appreciative inquiry is a good way to get more familiar with yourself, especially now that you know that you are, like all of us, composed of these various subpersonalities, each an expression of your basic needs. This is not a critique. You shouldn't be chastising yourself because your drive for autonomy is strong, at the expense of being as compassionate toward others as you should be, or being less curious, or less whatever. This is not an exercise in blame. Be grateful for each of the members of your Inner Family, but do get to know them. And a good way to start is by tracing their impact throughout your life. You may only now be aware that they are a part of you, but that doesn't mean they just appeared out of thin air. We talked earlier about the long evolutionary history behind these subpersonalities. You go back a long way! Start by understanding the role that these have had in steering your life's direction. Remember that Autonomy is often the part of one's personality that takes hold of that wheel.

The Four Questions You Need to Ask to Tune In to Your Inner Family and Decode Your Emotions

1. What role does this subpersonality play in my life, and how has it shaped me?
2. What story best captures its biggest contribution to my life?
3. On a scale of 1–10, how well are its needs being met today, and how important are those needs to my well-being?
4. What can I do to better meet the needs of this subpersonality?

1. What role does Autonomy play in my life, and how has it shaped me?

In order to better understand this part of you—the interplay between your genes and the experiences that have helped shape this member of your Inner Family—you need to know how Autonomy is working for you and just how much of a driving force it is (or isn't). So it's helpful to think about what it has done for you in your life.

Go back to your adolescence, because this is typically where the drive to self-actualize first shows up. Did you want to march to your own drummer in high school? As adolescents are often defined by their peer group, think about the kids you spent time with in high school. Were you part of the "in crowd" (to use a sixties term), or were you one of the "outliers" (a twenty-first-century term)?

Now follow yourself into your twenties. Did the autonomous drive play a role in how you chose your major in college, your first job, your career? Or did you change jobs or careers because you didn't have sufficient autonomy? Maybe this subpersonality didn't play as big a role for you as it did for others. That's okay. Each of the nine subpersonalities needs to be understood and appreciated, even the less vocal or dominant ones. It's important to value each one. After all, they're what makes you *you*.

2. What story best captures Autonomy's biggest contribution to my life?

These subpersonalities shouldn't be seen as abstractions, but as real driving forces that have an active presence in your life. Think about a time in your life when Autonomy had a big impact on you. Tell yourself a story. Better yet, tell it to a partner. (Describing your subpersonalities to another person, such as a spouse or a friend, is a great way to recognize and better understand your Inner Family.) Or write down your Autonomy story in a journal. Make it as detailed and as rich as you like. Just as the case study model in graduate school helps us to better understand principles of business and management, this personal "case study" approach is a useful way to see how the subpersonalities work for or against us.

Here's an example of an Autonomy story. It was related to Coach Meg recently by one of her clients, Eileen, now a fashion designer and a mother in her thirties. Eileen shared how Autonomy changed the direction of her life. Here's her story:

When I was in college, I wanted to go to Italy for a semester. I mean, why not? I was an art history major, and what country has more art and history than Italy? I loved the culture, the food. I'd watched every Italian movie I could get my hands on. I knew all the great Renaissance painters and sculptors. I figured this was the time in my life to do it. I felt a little confined in my private college. I'd spent the first two years taking required courses, many of which didn't seem relevant to what I wanted to do, which to be honest, I really wasn't sure of. Art history is not a very practical major, right? That's what my father kept reminding me of. So under a little pressure from him, I switched to art education at the beginning of my sophomore year. Still, a tough road. Jobs for an art teacher of any kind aren't easy to find.

I also knew teaching art wasn't really me. I was feeling kind of stifled. Education theory bored me, and when this opportunity came up to do a semester abroad in a place I'd always wanted to go, I had to say yes. I mean, Italy! It just seemed like a no-brainer.

My dad disagreed. He was concerned about my safety in a foreign country, concerned about me, a young American woman, traveling at a time of heightened international tensions. And I know he also thought that a trip to Italy might end up as a kind of prolonged vacation, like a semester-long spring break, except with me in Rome instead of Cancún. We argued on the phone. He finally said that he wouldn't pay for a semester abroad. I said, "Fine. I'll pay for it." Looking back, I know that this was me asserting my independence from him. But I was determined to do this. I really wanted to see with my own eyes the Sistine Chapel, the works of Leonardo da Vinci, and those of the other great masters. And yes, I admit, I did want to have an adventure overseas.

I worked two jobs that summer and saved up money, and in the second semester of my junior year, I took off for Italy. Right until the morning I left, my father refused to drive me to the airport, but in the end, he relented and gave me a big hug at the security gate.

I got to Italy, and the art history program at the sister college over there was terrific. I learned a lot about Renaissance art and became particularly intrigued by Caravaggio. But something else happened. During one of our side trips, this one to Milan, some of the other students and I got invited to attend a fashion show. It was my first exposure to these great designers and to this industry. I remember there was a cocktail reception, where we got to meet some of the designers. I began to see that what they did . . . fashion . . .

was really an artistic endeavor, and one in which Italy had helped set the standards, as much as it had in painting and sculpture five hundred years ago. I mean, I liked clothes. Lots of people do. But I'd never thought about them as art. The idea of being able to create my own designs, as opposed to being tied down to someone else's curriculum plan, was also appealing.

I came back at the end of that semester enchanted by Italy, by the glamorous fashion world, and with a new purpose. I shocked my father, the rest of my family and my friends, by announcing that I was changing my major to fashion design. Changing majors, transferring to another college . . . it was a lot of work. It also meant I would have to continue my college education for an extra semester, with me footing the bill for it. But it didn't matter. This was me. Designing dresses, suits, and outfits allowed me to express myself creatively, and in a way that everybody could see. I was creating things everybody needed, as opposed to doing paintings that no one would ever see.

That's kind of how it happened. I became a fashion designer, and I'm happy to be one. Oh, and one of my custom-made suits is hanging in my dad's closet. He wears it every Christmas Day, and when we're over there, he prompts everybody there to say how good it looks on him. And then he reminds everybody that his daughter designed it . . . because that's who she is.

A good story, right? And yet there's more to it. Eileen's Autonomy didn't live happily ever after. It rarely does. There was a reason Eileen came to Coach Meg, and we'll get into that soon. First, let's get back to those basic questions.

3. On a scale of 1–10, how well are Autonomy's needs being met today, and how important are those needs to my well-being?

You've looked in the rearview mirror, analyzed your own past. Now put yourself in the present. How well are your needs for autonomy being met today? How is this part of you, this member of your Inner Family, doing? Do you feel that you're free to march to your own drummer? Or maybe you're happy to fall in step with someone else's rhythm? The rhythm of your spouse, your partner, your boss?

Let's try to get a snapshot of this part of you:

A. *On a scale of 1–10, how important are Autonomy's needs to my well-being today?*

There's no right or wrong answer. Just bear in mind that the rating you give should be based genuinely on how driven you are by your need to be you. As Deci and Ryan tell us, the autonomous drive is an important motivation in all of us. But for some, it's *the* driving force. For you, maybe not. If your answer is a 5 or higher, you need to pay attention to it.

B. *On a scale of 1–10, how well are Autonomy's needs being met today?*

Do you feel you have the freedom to determine your own life's path, to make your own decisions? Do you have the freedom to express yourself and your abilities in a way that makes you feel genuine? The financially secure filmmaker or software designer or architect who is free to take on the projects he or she wants will probably rate this close to 10. Most of the rest of us, maybe a little lower.

The key is in the interplay of the two numbers from both 3a and 3b.

If your answer to both questions is 10, well, congratulations. You are apparently leading a very autonomous life. And how about if your answer is the opposite? Be careful here. If you rated the importance of the autonomous drive as a 2 and then gave a similar score to the question of how well your Autonomy's needs are being met, you may have to make some adjustments. Or to couch this in terms of the voices, they need to feel like they're being heard, not squelched, even if they are not the loudest ones in your Inner Family.

Keep in mind that even if someone is truly flourishing, they may not score high on question 3a for every subpersonality—because all of us have dominant parts of our personality—but they'll have mostly high scores for 3b. Even the less dominant subpersonalities require attention at some point.

Here's one more complicating factor: The scores change, especially for question 3b, over time.

The Time of Your (Autonomous) Life

There are several major life changes that affect our drive for autonomy.

The first, as we mentioned, is adolescence, when you're still developing a sense of self, trying to figure out who you are, and establishing the boundaries between you and your parents.

The second is when you start your adult life, which is one of the most frightening things you will do as a human being. It's a big world out there, it's very complicated, you're leaving the nest, and you don't have a clue. Whether that moment arrives when you go off to school or move out of the house or start your first full-time job, it's a critical point in life.

The next big life change comes a little later. You're in the midst of a career, and all of a sudden, you wake up and say, "This is not me. This is not what I want to do!" This doesn't happen to everyone, of course. But for so many of us, especially when Autonomy is a primary drive, it's an issue. You might be the lawyer, the businessperson, or the banker who wakes up one day and says, "I hate this!" It could be any career. (Coach Meg says that she's had teachers and physicians and even social workers who have come to her with this kind of dilemma.)

A common root of this discontentedness is a lack of autonomy. When kids refuse to eat their vegetables, resist going to bed when their parents ask them, or do the exact opposite of whatever their parents want them to do, they are often asserting their autonomy. A frustrated sense of autonomy is often what leads midlife adults into extramarital affairs, substance abuse, or other ill-advised behaviors. You're like a capped oil well, and the pressure of "I've gotta be me" just builds beneath the surface.

There's yet another point in your life when the autonomous voice cries out: when you're older. You may not be able to drive or live independently anymore. You have begun to lose the ability to do things that you could when you were young. When older adults say, "I'm not taking my medicine," or when they refuse even to consider moving to a senior residence or an assisted-living facility, we tend to think that they are being stubborn or cranky. But it's not just that. It's rebelliousness. It's defiance. It's their voice of Autonomy, still a strong part of their life force, being thwarted.

To get back to our self-assessment, at each stage of life, the score for question 3b ("How well are Autonomy's needs being met today?") will change based on our perceived sense of autonomy.

The rebellious teenager living at home and stuck in a classroom and in situations he or she has little say over (in part, we should add, because he or she may not yet be ready to make those kinds of decisions) is going to have a very high score for question 3a ("How important are Autonomy's needs to my well-being today?") and a very low one for 3b ("How well are Autonomy's needs being met today?")

That score may soar for individuals in their twenties, once they are living on their own and are comfortable with it, and—if they're fortunate—once they find themselves in a job in which they feel they are being themselves and are expressing their talents.

However, this score may change again. Consider the example of Eileen—our art history major who went to Italy against her father's wishes, only to find a new direction for herself there, in fashion design. As she related in her story, Eileen did indeed become a successful fashion designer. Along the way, she met a young buyer for a national chain of boutiques. They dated, fell in love, got married, and had a child. Eileen's score for Autonomy—which would have been a 9 or a 10 a few years ago—had plummeted to a 3 or a 4 by the time she came to see Coach Meg.

Why? Because she was a mom, yet another life stage when autonomy can be compromised. And like so many young moms with careers, Eileen had had to make some difficult decisions. In her case, she had taken a leave of absence from her design firm in order to care for her young son. She loved her child and wanted to be a responsible mom, but she couldn't help but feel that she now had less autonomy. How could she not?

This, too, will change as her son grows older.

The undulations and circumstances of life affect the degree to which our needs are being met. Coach Meg recommends checking in on these different subpersonalities every thirty days to see how they're doing.

For those with a low score for the question "How well are Autonomy's needs being met today?" the question then becomes, what do you do about that?

4. What can I do to better meet the needs of Autonomy?

The answer to bolstering a depleted sense of autonomy is obviously going to depend on one's circumstances. You can't tell that frustrated seventeen-year-old to quit school and leave home in order to better self-actualize. But when that teenager is planning his or her future, you can say that maybe going away to college would be a good idea, as opposed to living at home after he or she graduates high school.

Becoming more autonomous without making a drastic change in one's job or parenting situation usually involves finding ways to nibble around the edges, so to speak. In the case of the person feeling unfulfilled at work, it could be a hobby that provides him or her a greater degree of self-actualization. In the case of the mom, it could be taking on freelance or part-time work, which can be done while parenting is still the main focus. That's what Eileen did. After working with Coach Meg, Eileen decided to take on some part-time projects with her old design firm. This meant a couple of days commuting into the office, and that, in turn, meant hiring a babysitter. An added expense, yes, but a small price to pay for addressing a need that had driven Eileen since college and would most likely be a roaring force throughout her life.

Remember that everybody's got different ways and opportunities to express their autonomy. Think about yours. It could be something on the job. Perhaps you can identify, and suggest to your boss, a project that you could run on your own, with minimal supervision. Or it could be something you do on the weekends, on your own, or in your own spare time. Perhaps you want to climb a mountain. Train for a marathon or a triathlon. Become more autonomous by doing whatever you want to do that provides the beat to that drummer in you. It could be anything. Remember that unofficial national anthem of Autonomy, the old favorite that we mentioned, "I Gotta Be Me," sung by Sammy Davis Jr. Or maybe it's a new hit, "Roar," by Katie Perry.

CASE STUDIES:
Autonomy

Here are two case studies, both of which feature people who had challenges with the inner voice of Autonomy at different stages in their lives. Remember even the powerful voice of Autonomy is but one of nine members of your Inner Family. The first step toward better comprehending your emotions, taming the frenzy, and creating a life in which you are thriving entails getting in touch with all the members of your Inner Family. First, here's how that Roll Call sounded for one of Coach Meg's clients; the second case shows us how a patient of Dr. Eddie's was able to reclaim his autonomy.

Coach Meg: Laura, age twenty-four

When she came to Coach Meg, Laura was just a year or so out of college. A bright, talented young woman, she had a job in customer service with an online retailer, but her work entailed mostly handling computerized records. She didn't have any real interaction with customers. She came to Coach Meg because she felt like she needed more human contact in her job. She had worked on a lot of group projects as a management major during her college years, and she felt that she flourished in those situations. Leading a group, helping to make sure everyone had their assignments, reminding people of the big picture, and making sure everyone was pulling together—that's where she really felt her talents were.

In other words, she was a leader.

Coach Meg explained the Inner Family concept to Laura, taught her how to get to a state of mindfulness and, once Laura was in the moment, asked her to tap into each part of her personality. Here's what Laura reported when she asked each subpersonality to articulate its concerns:

Autonomy: "I'm not happy, because I'm not doing what I want to do. I've got a job. I'm making a living. But I'm not firing on all cylinders, I'm not doing what really gets me excited."

The Body Regulator: "Hang on! We've got a good job. We're saving up money. We have a good social life. Why do we want to rock the boat?"

Confidence: "I know that we liked those group projects in college, but this is real life now. I'm not sure if we can lead a project team or run a company."

The Creative: "We're not meeting my needs in this job. There is zero creativity in analyzing these customer service reports. So I'm with Autonomy on this!"

The Executive Manager: "We're good at this job, but I'll go along with whatever everyone else decides. Whatever we decide to do, I can make it work."

The Curious Adventurer: "This is all so boring. How about a little adventure? One of my friends moved to Colombia and said there are companies there that are looking for bright young Americans to step into management positions. Let's do it!"

The Relational: "I need to connect with people, and I like to help. It's pretty ironic that I'm in a customer-service position and I never get to talk to a customer."

The Standard Setter: "You don't know if you're ready to manage a team here, much less in South America. You think they'll listen to a twenty-four-year-old? As for Colombia, you barely speak Spanish. And don't forget, no matter what else anyone says about this job, we're good at it. We've gotten two raises since we've been here, and excellent performance evaluations."

The Meaning Maker: "Nobody has the perfect job in their first five years out of college. You want to travel? Fine. Travel. But let's be patient here. There's a lot to be said for the situation you're in right now."

Despite the mixed reactions, Laura felt better after going through the Roll Call. She and Coach Meg talked about the feedback she had received. Maybe the Body Regulator and the Standard Setter were right. Maybe an impetuous move wasn't the smartest play. Instead of quitting her job and heading for new horizons, she decided to explore opportunities *within* the company. In the meantime, at Coach Meg's suggestion, Laura looked around her community to find ways in which she could engage with those working toward a common purpose, so she could get the kind of human interaction and team experience she felt was so important to her. Watching the local news one night, she heard about a community group that was planning to clean up a local dump in order to make it into a nature preserve. They were looking for volunteers to work on a planning committee. Laura decided this would be a good way to connect with people and feel the satisfaction of working as part of a team effort and for a good cause. This turned out to be a wonderful experience for Laura, as she was eventually selected as chairperson of the committee.

About six months later, she was told about a management trainee job that had opened up in her company's home office in the Bay Area. Would she be interested? The job wasn't in South America, but it was on the other side of the country, and the Bay Area was a desirable place to live. Such a career move was also both an adventure and a stepping-stone to the kind of job she really wanted, the kind of work she felt she was best suited for. Laura said yes, got the job, and now lives, and is thriving, in Northern California.

Dr. Eddie: Patrick, age forty-nine

When Patrick, the CEO of a successful tech start-up, came to my office, he was in pain, not from any conflict among his inner voices or emotions, but from his knee. Yet I'd learned over the years that the way a patient dealt with a deteriorating joint or a broken bone was often closely linked to the inner frustration of a stunted personal need or drive.

Referred by his brother months ago, Patrick delayed taking the time from his busy schedule to evaluate his worsening knee pain until it became unbearable. When I entered the examination room, Patrick was sitting with his pant leg rolled up, working on his laptop computer and cell phone. He greeted me with a torrent of words, and at first, I wasn't even sure if he was talking to me or to someone on his Bluetooth . . . or both!

"I'm super busy with the planned launch of our new app, but my knee is really getting bad," Patrick said. "I can barely sleep, let alone do my cycling. I'm gaining weight from not exercising. You've got to help me. I don't know what to do. I can't seem to control this."

The diagnosis was not much of a mystery. Patrick's history of progressive pain, swelling, and stiffness, and the X-rays, clearly pointed to knee arthritis as the culprit. The challenge was to help Patrick gain some sense of control over the situation and support his strong sense of Autonomy within the setting of a generally paternalistic (and sometimes demeaning) medical visit.

"The good news is that my examination of your nerves, muscles, and all the other joints is normal," I informed him. "Everything points to osteoarthritis . . . the common wear-and-tear type . . . causing the pain in your right knee. There are some choices we should make about how you would like to proceed at this point." I ran down the list for him: pills to reduce the pain and swelling, icing, bracing, topical medications to rub on the knee, physical therapy to strengthen the leg, or possibly an injection to drain the extra fluid on the knee for quick relief. Losing a few pounds would also take some stress off the knee.

"What sounds best to you?" I asked. "How would you like to proceed?"

Patrick put aside his laptop and cell phone long enough to consider this. "Well," he replied, "I guess I feel better that you seem to know what's going on. But you're the doctor. Shouldn't *you* just tell *me* what to do?"

I had to stifle a smile. I'd heard this before. *Tell me what to*

do, Doctor. It's my body, it's my life, but you make the decision.
"This is not a life-threatening emergency," I explained to Patrick.
"So we have some time to make choices together about how to
proceed. You'll probably do best if you tell me which options
sound best to you. However, if you choose to have me make the
decisions about how to proceed, I can honor that."

Patrick pondered his alternatives. "Well, actually a biking
buddy of mine had the same problem and felt much better after
an injection," he said. "I don't mind needles, and I wouldn't mind
the quick relief. Then I could strengthen my knee in physical
therapy, and I can definitely lose the extra weight once I get
more active. The pills tend to upset my stomach, but that cream
to put on my knee sounds interesting."

"That sounds like a good plan," I replied. "If you don't get
some relief from the injection, the cream, and the physical therapy, we can try some other options."

Despite Patrick's compromised situation of severe pain and
perceived powerlessness, I wanted to do my best to support his
Autonomy. After what was no doubt a vociferous inner debate
among the members of his Inner Family, Patrick had initially offered to relinquish this power and have the doctor make the decisions for him, decisions that an assertive Autonomy might very
well have second-guessed later. However, with just a little push
back and acknowledgment that he was still in control of his own
destiny—knee-wise, at least—Patrick had quickly returned to his
more comfortable self-directed stance.

This is an example of how the Inner Family concept comes
into play in day-to-day situations and how those who recognize
its workings—in themselves and in others—are better at managing not only themselves but others, as well. The more straightforward aspect of this patient's care was managing his acute pain

and working to improve his function by choosing among several treatment options. But schooled in the ideas of this book, I recognized that by supporting Patrick's Autonomy, I could reduce his suffering from feeling out of control. Consequently, Patrick would likely be a more compliant patient. That, in turn, could directly affect his long-term prognosis as much as any pill or procedure. After all, he would be the one in charge of his daily habits to moderate his weight and maintain his strengthening exercises.

The injection and some physical therapy helped get the severe pain of his knee arthritis under control, and Patrick, with his Autonomy no doubt taking control, assisted by his Executive Manager, his Confidence, and his Standard Setter, took over the long-term tasks of losing weight and continuing his strengthening exercises. At this writing, he has lost fifteen pounds and is progressing nicely. Oh, and the app launched successfully, so much so that Patrick received some inquiries from potential buyers for his company. He considered those options just as he had his medical ones, and he decided he'd rather remain in control of his own business.

No surprise there.

THE BODY REGULATOR

You inhale. You exhale.

You sleep. You wake.

Your heart contracts as it pumps blood; then it relaxes as it fills with blood.

All the cyclical processes that keep us functioning are part of the oldest and most basic capacity that we possess: the Body Regulator.

Like the thermostat in your house, which adjusts automatically to the rise and fall of the indoor temperature, the Body Regulator quietly and efficiently goes about its business day after day, year after year. It thrives on rhythm and regularity.

As a member of your Inner Family, the Body Regulator is the one that functions like clockwork, following the same routine every day.

The Body Regulator likes stability.

The Body Regulator doesn't react well to change.

The Body Regulator plays it safe.

Indeed, homeostasis, the process by which organisms adjust

and adapt to the external environment in order to maintain internal stability, was part of the Body Regulator's primary evolutionary role. At the cellular level this is done by transporting selective materials in and out of the cell through a semi-permeable membrane, a process known as osmosis, in which water molecules are absorbed through the cellular membrane. The same safety mechanisms that nourish, maintain, and protect cells are built into the Body Regulator, which helps you maintain homeostasis in relation to your external environment. Sweating in the heat and shivering in the cold are just two examples of the Body Regulator making adjustments when those outside conditions change.

But the Body Regulator's drive for safety extends beyond the ambient air temperature. The voice that kept us alive when we were still evolving as a species now manifests itself as a voice of caution and self-preservation—along with being tied strongly to our physical needs and drives. This is the part of you that wants to stay home on Saturday night. The part that doesn't want to go to a party, board an airplane, take any kind of risk, or push any kind of boundary. Hence the Body Regulator often conflicts with the human drives that compel us to go places that aren't safe or stable. Such as the South Pole, the moon, or a new job in a new city.

The Body Regulator also plays a role in day-to-day decisions that can have important consequences. For example, some believe that if more people could just listen more closely to their Body Regulator, the country might not have an obesity epidemic. For most of us, the balance of appetite and satiety is finely tuned. Our bodies know when to stop eating, but factor in an overabundance of food, the need to soothe or reward ourselves, and other emotions associated with food, and that balance is thrown off. We end up eating more or different foods than our bodies need.

Those who have learned about the work of Abraham Maslow

will recognize the Body Regulator as representing the first two rungs of that psychologist's famous "hierarchy of needs"—a theory of motivation he first advanced in 1943. In Maslow's five-level hierarchy of needs, the biological needs—the need for food, water, and shelter—are considered the most basic and occupy the first level. On the second level is the need for safety. In contrast to the biological needs, writes communication theorist Em Griffin, the need for safety is mostly psychological. "Naturally we try to avoid a poke in the eye with a sharp stick," Griffin notes in his book *A First Look at Communication Theory*. "But once we've managed a certain level of physical comfort, we'll seek to establish stability and consistency in a chaotic world."

Given the chaos and the speed of change in today's world, that's a pretty tall order! The Body Regulator, then, encompasses a fairly wide range of needs and motivations: not only the primal urge to eat, but also a more advanced need, one that gives you the motivation, or the insight, to refuse to get in a car with a driver who's been drinking or to keep your personal credit card information off-line.

However, the voice of the Body Regulator, the embodiment of stability, is oftentimes easily drowned out. So we decide to get in that car, or we choose the cheeseburger with fries over the salad. Then again, strictly following the dictates of the Body Regulator can cause problems, too. As Griffin notes in his discussion of Maslow's safety need, "many adults go through life stuck on this level and act as if catastrophe will happen [at] any moment." In our conceptualization, the fear of making any kind of move, any kind of decision, can sometimes be attributed to a dominant Body Regulator, one that urges caution and adherence to safe, established practices at all costs.

But sometimes you need to take risks, or as the saying goes, break out of your comfort zone—the boundaries of which are established by your Body Regulator. Listen too much to this voice, and you might never leave the house. While it's sometimes a voice of wise caution, it can also be the voice of "No, you can't." "Don't do this." "Don't do that." Heed that voice consistently, and you'll end up doing nothing. Your personal and professional growth will be stunted. You're not likely to reach your full potential. You will be stuck in a rut.

More typical, though, is the person who's managed to tune out the Body Regulator, especially when it comes to his or her health. The body thrives on structured routine. If you're someone who is a regular exerciser, who follows a healthy diet, and who gets sufficient sleep, chances are you are pretty well tuned in to your Body Regulator, whether you know it or not. Because the body wants all that. It doesn't want to sit for hours on end. It needs to move. It wants good fuel, not just empty calories. It wants rest. It wants its balance. That's the Body Regulator.

It only makes sense to listen to this voice, which is essentially telling you what you need to do in order to maintain or improve your health. Yet it's so easy to ignore this voice. For people who overeat, people who let themselves go, people who are couch potatoes—the cries of the Body Regulator have been lost in the din of competing voices in what amounts to a vicious circle. "I see this a lot with people who are dealing with being overweight," says Coach Meg. "There is a fierce inner critic, the Standard Setter, saying angrily, 'How did you let yourself get like this?' and 'You're a failure.' Then their Confidence voice feels sad that it can't meet the inner standard. So then you have anger and sadness pushing you into a downward spiral, and what makes you feel better is a piece of cake! The last thing the Body Regulator wants you to have!" The Body Regulator just gets drowned out by the swirl of negative emotions.

A different response to the regulation of the body is found in the weekend warrior syndrome. "You get someone who doesn't exercise during the week, and they overexercise during the weekend. They train through pain. They overdo it." This approach to exercise entails ignoring the voice of the Body Regulator, too, which, in this case, would be offering the kind of common-sense advice you've read in fitness magazines: start slowly, don't overdo it, make sure to hydrate, and so forth. But for these individuals, the voices of Confidence and the Standard Setter are bellowing, and theirs is a different tune. "It might be the macho message of 'I have to prove myself,'" Coach Meg says, "or it might be the Standard Setter saying, 'You have to do better.'"

Again, the Body Regulator's voice loses the competition for attention.

So are you listening to your Body Regulator? What kind of role is it playing in your life? Is it part of the problem or part of the solution? We'll look at case studies of each scenario, but first, we invite you to ask yourself the four questions discussed in chapter 4, this time with your Body Regulator in mind:

1. What role does the Body Regulator play in my life, and how has it shaped me?
2. What story best captures the Body Regulator's biggest contribution to my life?
3. On a scale of 1–10, how well are the Body Regulator's needs being met today, and how important are those needs to my well-being?
4. What can I do to better meet the needs of the Body Regulator?

Let's take them one by one.

1. What role does the Body Regulator play in my life, and how has it shaped me?

If you're in good health, if you're exercising regularly, sleeping well, and eating the right foods, the Body Regulator is playing a positive role in your life. If you're out of shape, if you're over-weight, if your doctor's been telling you that you need to make changes to your lifestyle but you haven't really responded to that call to action, well, then, the Body Regulator's voice may be on mute in your Inner Family.

2. What story best captures the Body Regulator's biggest contribution to my life?

Remember that while the Body Regulator may be a need we have in common with single-cell organisms, it's not as if it is simply a primitive instinct or an unintelligent entity. It can help you do more than remember to breathe! Example: While the motivation to do so might have come from elsewhere, the Body Regulator probably helped you train for and complete your first half mara-thon or triathlon or successfully adopt a vegan diet. Maybe it's this voice of stability and safety that kept you from impetuously taking that job offer on the other side of the country last year. Oh, it sounded great and exciting. After all, it was a new start-up. But the Body Regulator pointed out the stability and security of your current job. It might have seemed like you made a dull decision at the time, but not when that new start-up went belly-up after just six months, which would have left you unemployed and three thousand miles from home, had you thrown caution to the wind and taken that job. You can thank your Body Regulator—which is always looking out for you—that you didn't!

3. On a scale of 1–10, how well are the Body Regulator's needs being met today, and how important are those needs to my well-being?

If the answers to both questions are a 5 or below, working on meeting the Body Regulator's needs would do a lot to improve your overall thriving. (And you may want especially to work on heeding the Body Regulator and meeting its needs because this subpersonality could directly affect your health!)

4. What can I do to better meet the needs of the Body Regulator?

While this isn't a "how to get in shape" book, it's worth noting that a major study conducted by researchers at Johns Hopkins University in 2013 showed that adhering to four behaviors can dramatically increase your chances of leading a longer, healthier life:

- ✦ Don't smoke.
- ✦ Maintain a healthy weight.
- ✦ Engage in regular physical activity.
- ✦ Make healthy food choices (the subjects in this nationwide study followed a Mediterranean diet).

Chances are, those findings merely reinforce much of what your Body Regulator has been telling you. These are the kinds of behaviors it craves (maybe even more than you crave sugar or having your feet up on the recliner!). If you are not already engaging in such lifestyle behaviors, the changes you make in this area would enable you to meet the needs of the Regulator, which would reciprocate in kind. This subpersonality's need for routine could help you in your efforts to get into a regimen of exercise and healthy eating and to sustain the new healthier habits.

CASE STUDIES:
The Body Regulator

COACH MEG: Bobby, age thirty-nine

When Coach Meg met Bobby, a professional firefighter, he lumbered into her office, sipping on a can of diet soda. As they shook hands in greeting, she watched as her hand was swallowed up by his.

"He was a big guy," recalls Coach Meg.

Bobby knew that his size was part of his problem. He came to Coach Meg after he had been diagnosed as prediabetic. Bobby, who stood six feet two inches tall, had weighed around 180 pounds in high school, where he'd been a standout halfback on the football team. He had gone into the navy after high school, then had worked in construction for a few years, before becoming a firefighter. That was when his weight began soaring. "They talk about the freshman fifteen in college," Bobby said. "Well, they have the same thing in the firehouse." Especially in Bobby's firehouse. "I had an old-time captain who loved to fry up potatoes and bacon. And, boy, they tasted good."

After a few years, his weight had ballooned to three hundred pounds. With two young children to look after, Bobby knew he had to start taking his health seriously. Changes were needed. The diagnosis of prediabetes finally lit the fire. Bobby and his physician knew that weight loss was a complex issue. Bobby had tried a few diets in the past and had failed. This time he was determined to get it right. His physician suggested working with a health coach to help make the changes in his lifestyle that he needed in order to shed his extra weight, and with the encouragement of his wife, who'd been on him about his weight for a couple of years, Bobby decided to give it a go.

After explaining the Inner Family concept to Bobby, Coach Meg suggested that he do a Roll Call. He was dubious.

"All these voices in my head . . . you want me to tune in to them?" he asked skeptically.

Coach Meg explained that they weren't voices from the beyond, but that they were part of the internal monologue he had with himself all day long. "It's all you," she said. "But just different aspects of your personality, each representing different drives and needs."

Bobby was still skeptical, until he found himself articulating things that clearly bespoke some different points of view and mixed emotions within him. And they revealed a tug-of-war within over what it took to maintain his health.

Autonomy: "I'm a guy. I want to eat what I want to eat, and it's not tofu."

Confidence: "I need my three squares. You can't get through a fire on lettuce and cucumber sandwiches. Besides, I'm not sure I can change the way I eat at this point in my life."

The Creative: "I've come up with some pretty creative solutions to stuff at home. I can probably do the same here. I like to cook. Maybe it would be fun to learn some new recipes for things that might be better for me."

The Curious Adventurer: "I read that this kale stuff is good for the brain. I need quick reflexes when we're on a call . . . so maybe I should be thinking about this a little different. I'm probably in a rut with this stuff I've been eating for years. Maybe I'd feel better."

The Executive Manager: "All this fried stuff, these heavy meals, makes me sluggish. And I'm winded just taking the stairs. I can't do my job and meet my responsibilities at home if I'm walking around tired all the time."

The Relational: "I like being one of the guys, and mealtime is when we hang out. I can't be the only one eating steamed broccoli while they're digging into fried chicken. I'm going to have to find someone else who wants to change their diet, too."

The Standard Setter: "I saw a picture of myself from high school the other day. I was lean and mean back then. Man, I've turned into a fat middle-aged guy. It's kind of depressing."

The Body Regulator: "You're killing me! I've been saying all along that this whole schedule is throwing me off. It's hard enough with the shifts we have to do. But when you're out of shape and tired all the time that just makes it impossible for us to function."

The Meaning Maker: "As a lieutenant, I'm expected to be a leader in the firehouse. That captain who mentored us and taught us how to cook? He was a great guy, but you remember he had a heart attack at age fifty-one and had to retire on disability? This is an opportunity to be a *real* leader, to change the culture. And to make sure your girls have a dad who can walk them down the aisle someday, not sit in the church in a wheelchair."

When the Roll Call was done, the usually affable Bobby was somber, his head down. Sometimes it's one voice that makes all the difference. In this case, it was listening to the Meaning Maker that really compelled Bobby to start paying attention to the Body Regulator. Hearing himself talk about his responsibilities as a leader, about ensuring the health of the men in his firehouse, not to mention his responsibilities to his family, really seemed to hit him. "I asked him what he was thinking about," Coach Meg says. "He replied, 'I need to step up here. I need to show my guys we have to change things. And the change has to start with me.'"

Bobby started making things happen fast. He invited a dietitian to come in and give a talk at his firehouse. He began going for morning walks with his wife. He instituted a weight-loss challenge at the firehouse, with the net proceeds going to charity. When one of his men suggested cycling together, Bobby embraced the idea. He bought a bike and organized some group rides. A year later he did his first century, a one-hundred-mile bike ride. By then he was thirty pounds lighter, and his blood sugar and A1C levels were normal. He had reversed his prediabetes, had established himself as a real leader in the firehouse, and had made his family, himself, and that part of him known as the Body Regulator very happy.

Dr. Eddie: Rose, age fifty-eight

As you've read, the Body Regulator is the prime voice representing the physical needs of the body. As a physician specializing in musculoskeletal care, I routinely see patients for whom this voice is rarely heard: it's weak, unattended to, sometimes even mute.

Until something goes really wrong, and then it starts to scream.

Not listening to our Body Regulator leads us to eat when we are not hungry, to stay up when we are tired, and to sit when we should be moving. We end up overweight, sleep deprived, and out of shape. Such is the case with Rose, a fifty-eight-year-old executive assistant, who is overweight, inactive, and chronically fatigued from getting less than six hours of sleep each night. She presents at my office periodically to give voice to her Body Regulator when, after being ignored for long periods of time, it finally has no choice but to bellow, "My back hurts so much that I can't even sit at work."

The root cause of Rose's back pain is stress from carrying too much weight around her middle and having too little strength in her core muscles. As I have done in the past, during one office visit, I gently implored her to eat smaller quantities of healthier foods, to start a strengthening program for her abdomen and back, and to get up and walk periodically during her workday to avoid the back pain. However, I also offered the "quick fix" of medication and an injection to quiet the pain and get Rose back to work. Unfortunately, she has used such brief respites from pain as an opportunity to put her Body Regulator back on mute once again. Of course, I was wise to this by now.

"Rose, the medication is not a long-term solution," I told her. "What you really need is to start modifying your diet and doing some of the exercises I've prescribed for you."

"Oh, thank you, Dr. Phillips," said ever-polite Rose. "I know you're right. You always give me good advice."

"Yes," I wanted to shout at her. "And my advice is overruled by your Inner Family!" But I couldn't really get mad at her. Frustrated by her inability to break the cycle of dysfunction, yes, but angry, no. Because truth be told, most of us struggle with our Body Regulator in some aspect or another.

You might assume that it would be somehow easier for me as a physician to pay close attention to my own Body Regulator. Indeed, while going through the rigors of medical school and residency training, I treated my health as a "commodity" that I could spend down like a savings account. In a sense I was constantly calculating how little sleep, exercise, and healthy food would suffice and still allow me to perform on exams and treat patients efficaciously. Whenever I exceeded my own physical limits, my Body Regulator would loudly announce that I had stepped over the line, reporting that I was run-down and feeling cranky. At one low point I caught pneumonia during my internship. As I look back, I realize that the first inner voice that I routinely consulted was my Body Regulator. For me, it may indeed be the clearest and loudest voice when I am sick and in pain, as it probably is for others.

As I progressed into medical practice and became more involved in lifestyle medicine, I evolved to the point where I asked my Body Regulator not just how I could avoid being sick but what I could do to feel more energetic, productive, and happy. Over time listening to the voice of my Body Regulator helped me realize that heeding its call for adequate rest, good food, and sufficient physical activity not only helped me avoid illness but also resulted in improved energy, a brighter outlook, more productivity, and less pain.

I now offer this perspective of expanding wellness, vibrancy, and joy of life to my patients. I teach Rose and my other patients to listen to their Body Regulator, not only to quiet their back pain and treat other ailments but also to achieve increasingly higher levels of wellness. The conversation continues.

6

CONFIDENCE AND
THE STANDARD SETTER

Believe in yourself! Have faith in your abilities! Without a humble but reasonable confidence in your own powers you cannot be successful or happy."

Those are the stirring words of Norman Vincent Peale, the apostle of self-affirmation. His book *The Power of Positive Thinking* has sold more than seven million copies in fifteen languages since it was first published in 1952, according to Important Books, the current publisher of this landmark title.

Peale, who died in 1993, at the age of ninety-five, was what journalists would call "a quote machine"—perhaps not surprisingly, since he started his career as a newspaper reporter in the Midwest. But later he became a minister and was famous for his sermons on the importance of a positive outlook toward life. Although his mid-twentieth-century message may seem quaint in the cynical age in which we now live, his pithy sayings remain powerful and, thanks to the Internet, reverberate to this day.

What's notable about the particular quote at the beginning of this chapter (which often shows up as number one on the Norman Vincent Peale hit parade), is that he is really talking about two related traits: confidence and self-esteem.

They're distinct and yet related. They're also both important members of your Inner Family. Of course, self-esteem goes by a different name, the Standard Setter, which also plays the role of inner critic and judge.

Because of their close association, we will look at both Confidence and the Standard Setter in this chapter to help you better recognize their relationship, their different voices, and their different points of view in your ongoing internal dialogue.

CONFIDENCE

Confidence, narrowly defined, is your assessment of whether you can succeed at the task at hand. You can widen the lens to consider your confidence in all small and large life domains, from "Can I fix this leaky faucet on my own, or do I need to call a plumber?" to "Can I live a life of rich meaning, purpose, contentment, and joy?"

Let's go back to the psychologists Deci and Ryan and their self-determination theory. The theory asserts that competence is one of the three most compelling human psychological needs. And it's often flying high in your earliest years. Most children are brimming with confidence. That's because they're learning to walk, learning to talk, learning to read—and they're *doing* it. They're getting better. They're growing, getting stronger, gaining competencies. That's not to say that children don't hit bumps on the developmental road and don't have setbacks. Of course they do. But just by the very nature of growing up, they are gaining confidence. After all, they start with a blank slate.

As life goes on, we become more confident about our abilities on a wider range of things. The child can learn to speak; the adult can learn to speak in public. The child can learn to walk; the adult runs his or her first 5K or marathon. As you get older, however, it becomes a mixed bag. The sixty-five-year-old professional has probably gained a great deal of confidence in his or her ability to deal with issues related to work and career. But at the same time, physical abilities, and sometimes such things as the ability or willingness to change with the times or adopt new technologies, may have diminished.

Clearly, whether we are young, old, or middle-aged, confidence is a guiding force in our lives. Our confidence is what gets us a job, gives us the courage to enter into a relationship, and enables us to move out of our parents' house and into our first apartment or home. (And a lack of confidence, on the other hand, may keep us from doing all of these things.)

Confidence is talking to you all the time, not just during the pivotal moments of your life. It's about throwing a baseball, preparing a meal, changing a flat tire. All the skills that we build in life are driven in part by this subpersonality, which wants to get better and develop competence. Humans love to be competent, love to prove their competence, love to tell (or, better, show) people how competent they are. That's why we love telling people what to do, even though the Autonomy part of us hates being told what to do. We love to do what we dislike being done to us. Now, that's cognitive dissonance.

Competence is an important word when discussing Confidence.

In fact, Richard Schwartz, creator of the Internal Family Systems model, suggests that this subpersonality could be labeled as such, because our confidence emerges from our competence. One can have the drive to be confident, and confidence comes from being competent. (On the flip side, the drive to be competent generates the competence that gives one confidence.)

SELF-ESTEEM AND THE STANDARD SETTER

Self-esteem derives from one's assessment of one's self-worth and from the validation, respect, and appreciation that one enjoys. Am I worthy or valuable as a human being? Am I respected by myself and others? Am I good enough? For younger people, self-esteem hinges to a significant degree on what others think of them. Their value is determined by the opinions of their parents, teachers, and, maybe most of all, peers. The more mature we get, the less preoccupied we are with what other people think, although it doesn't go away entirely for most of us. We become more concerned with what we think of ourselves. This is the part of you that decides where to set the bar and what is good enough, and then evaluates your accomplishments—or your perceived lack thereof—against an inner standard or an "internalized outer" one (meaning your evaluation of yourself is based on your perception of the way in which others, such as family, peers, or society, evaluate you).

The voice of the Standard Setter can be momentarily or consistently harsh and unforgiving: "I've never amounted to anything." "I'm a disappointment to myself." "I'm a failure." On the other hand, it can also be sycophantic, telling you what you want to hear—or perhaps what you've been told by well-meaning people. In other words, your self-esteem can be too high. Some believe that this is the case with a significant proportion of our society today.

A 2013 BBC story, "Does Confidence Really Breed Success?" reported on a study of American college freshmen that examined their confidence and self-esteem relative to their actual achievements. The study looked at the annual results of the American Freshman Survey—taken by about nine million college students since 1966—and found that over the past few decades, there has been a steep rise in those who consider themselves "above average" in their academic abilities, their drive to achieve, and their self-confidence.

Objective measures, however, present a different picture. For example, while students who took the survey were increasingly likely to consider themselves gifted writers, tests have showed that the writing ability of college students has actually gone down since the 1960s. Another statistic the researchers cited is that the amount of study time reported by most college freshmen has declined. Yet in that same period there has been a corresponding rise in the number of students who claim to have a drive to succeed.

Granted, the amount of time spent with one's nose in the books is not always synonymous with success, but still these results suggest a disconnect with reality. "What's really become prevalent over the last two decades is the idea that being highly self-confident . . . loving yourself, believing in yourself . . . is the key to success," said Jean Twenge, lead author of the study, who was quoted in the BBC story. "Now the interesting thing about that belief is it's widely held, it's very deeply held, and it's also untrue."

Untrue? The idea that high self-esteem is a prerequisite for success? Norman Vincent Peale must be spinning in his grave.

Then again, perhaps due to the influence of apostles of positivity like Peale and others, self-esteem did get too much emphasis, and the pendulum swung too far, engendering the notion that believing in one's competence and value was the key to success and to solving all life's problems. But now, some say that pendulum may be swinging too far back in the opposite direction. Self-esteem remains a primary human need—not the only one, of course, but one that should not be dismissed because American college students seem to have a bit too much of it or because it may not always correlate with success. Thriving comes through a healthy balance, a meeting of most or all our needs. Achieving that balance requires an understanding of how these needs work and how they manifest themselves in our lives.

Certainly it will be interesting to see if the millennials—whose self-esteem has so famously been pumped up, as they have been fed the "you're so special" sauce by their parents since childhood—change their perceptions of their self-worth as they grow older. If they're like preceding generations, they will. The fortunes of life alone, alas, will no doubt make a dent.

"I think self-esteem is the place where we see how evolved we are," says Coach Meg. "You go from defining your worth based on what others think when you're young to defining your worth based on your appraisal of your contributions and achievements when you're an adult." That inner critic can be very judgmental. And for different reasons. For young people, that inner critic is often most critical about social status, physical appearance, and hipness—or their perceived lack of these. For older professional men and women, that inner critic is often questioning the person's performance, contribution to the greater good, and status. Regardless of what's being scrutinized, our Standard Setter—essentially, the voice of our self-esteem—can be quite harsh. It's the part of us that gets angry at ourselves for screwing up, and it can be a dominant voice for many people who regret missed opportunities and poor decision making.

"I should have accepted that job offer two years ago."
"I should have married so-and-so when I had the chance."
"I should have started investing earlier."

It's these regrets, the "what should have beens," that often bring people to a coach. "'Shoulda, coulda, woulda.' This is a common refrain," says Coach Meg. "As a coach, I want to get people to find a bit more contentment. Instead of 'How good am I?' we try to focus on 'How can I get better?'"

Maybe it means working a little harder or smarter next time or being better prepared. Maybe it means negotiating a bit with the Standard Setter, reminding this part of you that is the demanding taskmaster that those harsh judgments are often counterproductive, as they not only diminish self-worth but erode confidence, leaving you feeling depleted. And without confidence, you can't achieve, which, after all, is what the Standard Setter is concerned about. That's how these two subpersonalities, Confidence and the Standard Setter, although separate, influence each other.

Let's talk a little bit more about the subpersonality Confidence. In "Overcome the Eight Barriers to Confidence," an article published in 2014 in the *Harvard Business Review*, Harvard Business School professor Rosabeth Moss Kanter defines *confidence* as "an expectation of a positive outcome." "It is not a personality trait; it is an assessment of a situation that sparks motivation," she writes.

This view seems to suggest that the voice of Confidence is

motivated and is not afraid to act appropriately or rationally in a given situation, even when there are pressures to do otherwise. However, one's situational assessment of competence isn't always accurate; one can overestimate or underestimate competence, which is something to watch out for. The following are examples of both.

Some friends of yours at work invite you to take a boot camp class with them. It's a pretty high-intensity class. They've been doing it for months . . . but they think it would be a lot more fun if you came along after work.

The voice of (Over) Confidence says, "You'll be fine! So what if you've never taken an indoor cycling class? You know how to ride a bike, and you're not totally out of shape. And look at these people in the class. They don't look like superathletes. You're every bit as good as them. Don from Accounting is ten years older than you, for heaven's sake! And Betty . . . she's in the class. Didn't she have back problems at one point? If they can do it, you can, too."

You listen to (Over) Confidence, and take the class. It's way more demanding than you expected. You try to keep up with the rest of the class—especially Don and Betty—and you're so trashed that at the end, you don't even bother stretching. The next day, you wake up hobbling. You've injured your Achilles tendon, your doctor tells you, but you know that what got you was an acute case of overconfidence. Now you can't exercise at all for a few weeks. Thanks a lot, Confidence!

The voice of (Under) Confidence reacts differently to the offer from your office mates to join them for the boot camp class. "Are you crazy? You're not ready for this class. You've been walking the dog, which is certainly good physical activity, but it's not high-intensity training. Forget about Don and Betty. Matt in Marketing is in that class, and he was a lacrosse player in college or something like that. Diana did a triathlon. Look at her. . . . She's totally toned. You're not ready to be in the same exercise class with her. Maybe if you put a little effort into it and gradually build up your wind. But certainly not now."

You end up not taking the class, and feeling miserable about the fact that you're not in shape. But at least you don't get hurt! If you heed the advice of (Under) Confidence—or perhaps it should be called (Realistic) Confidence—you don't have to nurse an injured Achilles tendon.

If you did take the boot camp class, perhaps the Standard Setter had something to do with it. Perhaps pressure to keep up with your office mates triggered (Over) Confidence: "You wimp. Of course you should be able to do the boot camp class." And if you passed on the class, perhaps the harsh assessments of the Standard Setter led to (Under) Confidence: "The last time you did a new workout, you couldn't walk for a week, you loser." An objective, encouraging Standard Setter might help Confidence be realistic and might simply challenge you to build up your fitness, arguing that by taking some introductory group exercise classes and modifying your diet, you could drop a few pounds, increase your cardiovascular conditioning, and then at some point join your fit friends from work in the class, without feeling embarrassed or out of place . . . and without hurting yourself.

Generally, as your confidence grows, so, too, does your self-esteem. Again, these two separate voices, Confidence and the Standard Setter, are mutually influential.

How do you ascertain what Confidence and the Standard Setter are saying? Let's ask our four questions, this time with these two subpersonalities in mind.

1. What roles do Confidence and the Standard Setter play in my life, and how have they shaped me?

To some extent, this depends on where you are in life. As we've seen, confidence and self-esteem fluctuate and evolve throughout childhood. After that flurry of confidence building during the blank slate of childhood, adolescents and young adults often lack confidence, because they have little yet to base it on. How can you be confident about doing anything that is considered part of adult life—managing money and credit cards, holding a job, maintaining a relationship—when you are eighteen years old? Adolescents' and young adults' confidence can be shaky, and their self-esteem is oftentimes lowered by this wobbly confidence. (But as noted, some research now suggests that the self-esteem of younger people has been pumped up a little too much.)

A good laboratory in which to see how confidence and self-esteem can be built among young people is the U.S. military, particularly the United States Marine Corps (USMC). The methods may be harsh (although not as much as in the past), but the simple fact that the USMC, year after year, takes thousands of young American men and women of varying backgrounds and abilities and produces physically fit, disciplined, and motivated warriors at the end of the training is proof that they understand something about how to bolster confidence. It's doubtful that many young marines have a timid voice of Confidence—although that was probably not the case when they first stepped off the bus at the marine corps training bases at Parris Island, South Carolina, or Camp Pendleton, California.

What role does the Standard Setter play for young marines while their confidence is being built in boot camp? A young marine might have a role model, such as the Navy SEAL sniper in the 2014 film *American Sniper*, a heroic marine from Iwo Jima whom he or she has read about, or perhaps a parent or an older sibling who served. Through this example, the young marine can be driven to achieve and accomplish something equivalent. This drive to achieve comes from the Standard Setter. This can be a healthy push, but if it's too strong and judgmental, the individual may feel browbeaten. The interplay between the voice of Confidence and that of the Standard Setter is a delicate one, then. The Standard Setter is continuously negotiating with Confidence and perhaps pushing it beyond the comfort zone.

For adults in the corporate world, Confidence might be embodied in the colleague who has no problem standing up and voicing her opinions in a meeting. Or telling your best client that what he is asking for is unrealistic. Or diving into the new software, which has changed the look of your computer screen and almost everything you do with it, without a tutorial or even any whining! Here, too, the inner negotiations continue. It takes healthy self-esteem to have the confidence to do those things—but the Standard Setter shouldn't be shaken to the core if the recommendations voiced at the meeting are not acted upon, if the client insists on what he wants, or if the attempts to master the new software result in a blank computer screen.

2. What stories best capture Confidence's and the Standard Setter's biggest contributions to my life?

Was it the promotion you accepted, even though it meant taking on a whole lot of new responsibilities and mastering new skills? Was it when you dared to ask the man or woman of your dreams for their hand in marriage? Or said yes to the person who did the asking? Was it when you agreed to run the charity 10K—and then proudly displayed your finisher's medal on your mantelpiece? Was it when you agreed to assume the PTA presidency or teach the Sunday school class at your church?

All these endeavors, to some degree, involve risk. You have to take some risks to become more competent and confident and thereby to build self-esteem.

Confidence is a voice that coaches are often called upon to bolster. "Coaches help people build competence and confidence by encouraging an experimental mind-set that is more concerned with learning than with judging success and failure," says Coach Meg. "Or we help people calibrate realistic goals, so that they get to stretch their abilities a little, but not too much."

The Standard Setter can be a source of perseverance when Confidence is struggling: it can get someone through a tough project or situation. It asks Confidence to get up after each failure or setback. There may be occasions when it pushes too hard, is too tough a taskmaster, leading to failure and bruising Confidence. Striking the balance between striving and having confidence in our ability is something we do in every task and project. It's an ongoing dialogue, a part of every story about Confidence.

Confidence is built well by taking small steps. The Standard Setter can be helpful in getting you to take that first step; and it can be a beneficiary of your success, as demonstrated competence can also reinforce or bolster self-esteem, as well as confidence. But the Standard Setter can also be an obstacle. "Why bother?" the Standard Setter with low self-esteem might say when you're about to take that first step in learning or attempting something new. "You're not good enough to do that, anyway." Competence comes from learning and experience. Want to build confidence? Keep stretching yourself. Learn new things. Experiment with new ways of doing things. It's a growth mind-set. "Kids take small steps, baby steps," says Coach Meg. "Then they add to them gradually. This is how kids build confidence, and it works just as well for adults."

Whether you're learning how to speak in public or learning how to grow a garden in your backyard, confidence building follows the same formula: Establish your goal and devise a reasonable plan to meet that goal. Then take the first step. Assess it. Reflect on it. Then, based on what you've learned, take the next step. Step-by-step, you build competence. Step-by-step, confidence grows. And as an additional bonus, self-esteem grows, too.

3. On a scale of 1–10, how well are Confidence's and the Standard Setter's needs being met today, and how important are those needs to my well-being?

Confidence is often the deciding factor in whether you do something or not. The life of inaction is very often led by the person with little confidence. When you lack confidence, you procrastinate. You are reluctant to step up and take the bull by the horns. While overconfidence can be a problem, too, in order to thrive, coaches encourage their clients to raise their Confidence score to around 7 or 8 for a particular task. Certainly, above 5*.

Yes, that's an asterisk you see next to that number. It's there because unlike with some of the other subpersonalities, the Confidence score often depends on the particular domain. There is no number that is applicable to all aspects of your life. You might be confident about your abilities as a parent, but not as a professional. You might be confident that you can fix something that's broken, but you could never get up in public and speak. You could be confident about golf but lousy at tennis. And maybe you're right about that! (Although, of course, it doesn't mean you can't improve your tennis game and thus build your confidence in that area, if you so choose.)

You're a mixed bag. This score is a composite of all domains of your life. So when you consider your Confidence score, it might be useful to consider which domain you're talking about.

What about the Standard Setter in all this? As noted before, sometimes this voice is hard to please, as we are always comparing ourselves to others, showing ourselves where we are falling short, and pointing out where we are not good enough. Ideally, the Standard Setter applies just enough pressure, without becoming nasty and judgmental. As you have seen, self-esteem is often closely linked to confidence, so it's probably a safe bet that your score for the Standard Setter will be closely linked to that for Confidence.

4. What can I do to better meet the needs of Confidence and the Standard Setter?

Learn more. Experience more. Try more. But do it in small steps, so that Confidence isn't anxious or overwhelmed. Try not to judge yourself too harshly along the way. If you encounter roadblocks, work around them and keep moving forward. As Frederich Nietzsche said, "What doesn't kill you makes you stronger."

Also, remember Confidence's connection to the Standard Setter: the more confidence you have, the greater your self-esteem is likely to be. As we have said, Confidence and the Standard Setter impact each other to a great degree. In our two case studies, you will see examples of how that happens. Sometimes these two subpersonalities reinforce one another, but not always. Notice also how addressing one can often help with the other.

Life from start to finish is about becoming more competent and confident as a human being. And so every day you can set out to get a little better in some domain or some aspect of your life. It could be just learning how to make a better breakfast. Or how to be more assertive on the job. Or how to do home repairs. Or anything. Pick one area and focus on it. Confidence will come. In the next section, we'll show you how.

BUILDING CONFIDENCE STEP-BY-STEP

It starts with building *competence*.

"One of the main things we do as coaches is help people to build confidence by gradually improving competence," says Coach Meg.

Want to bolster your competence, and in turn your confidence, in any aspect of your life? Take these steps.

- ◆ *Find a role model:* What are you looking to do? To play the piano or start a business or become less shy in social situations? Whatever your goal, find someone whom you can relate to and who already demonstrates competence in that area. Learn about this person and how he or she does it and, if possible, observe this person in action.

- *Stretch a little, but not too far:* Don't try to play a Beethoven sonata your second time in front of the keyboard. And remember, a successful business is not built in a day—or even in a year. It, too, takes time, as does getting more comfortable around others. Figure out the first step; make it small, reasonable, perhaps measurable.

- *Have a mind-set of learning, not judgment:* Take that first step. It's just an experiment. (Indeed, all of life can be seen as one big experiment.) See what happens. It may get you exactly where you want to go. It may not. Either way, don't judge yourself. Don't let a critical Standard Setter dominate the internal discussion. Unpack and harvest the learning from your experience as you plan your next step.

- *Look for opportunities to improve:* Design experiences that build mastery. Ask for advice from your role model. Seek out instruction, if needed, either from teachers or coaches or health professionals or reading material. And whenever you can, practice!

- *Take a couple more steps . . . and build on them:* Incorporate what you've learned from your first step and your opportunities to improve, and then take another step. And another. With each one, review and reflect on what you've learned. Build on those steps.

- *Be optimistic:* It may take time, but if your goal is realistic, and you're determined and kind to yourself, you will get there. In the process, you'll boost your confidence and self-esteem!

CASE STUDIES:
Confidence and the Standard Setter

COACH MEG: Jason, age twenty-one, and Elizabeth, age fifty-two

Jason, a junior in college, and his mother, Elizabeth, a successful attorney, came to see Coach Meg together, an unusual occurrence, but not unheard of in coaching circles.

Elizabeth and her husband had gone along with Jason when, in his freshman year, he told them he was majoring in education. But now, two years later, they were hoping that he'd rethink his original plan. They were hoping he would follow in their footsteps and go to law school. Jason's dad even dreamed of his son eventually coming to work as a junior partner in his firm.

Jason wasn't interested in law school—and if anything, his classes in education and a semester of student teaching in an inner-city school had reaffirmed his ambition to become a teacher. "It's a noble calling," he reminded his parents during one discussion. "The country needs good teachers, and I could do a lot more to help society in that job than as a corporate lawyer."

"Be practical," his parents told him. "Getting a good-paying teaching position is going to be hard, and who knows where you might have to live." They urged him to take the LSATs.

This led to further heated debates over what was a meaningful career.

While his parents respected Jason's ability to make a decision, Elizabeth told Coach Meg, "My husband's attitude is, 'If we're paying his tuition, don't we deserve at least a say?'"

Hence, the visit to Coach Meg for some coaching.

After explaining the Inner Family concept, Meg invited Jason to do a Roll Call, while his mom sat and listened:

Autonomy: "I'm very proud of my mom. She's been very successful. But I don't necessarily want to be like her. She works seventy hours a week, and it seems like she has a lot of stress in her job, which distracts her from enjoying the weekend. The money's good, but I don't care as much about money. I'm a different person, and I have different goals."

The Body Regulator: "I like outdoor sports, and I especially love going hiking and rock climbing on weekends. I know that's out if I become a lawyer. Those junior associates work Saturdays and sometimes Sundays. That doesn't sound good for your body or your mind."

Confidence: "I've listened to my mom and dad my whole life. I see how they have to think as lawyers. I just don't think I could do that as well as they do. I just don't have . . . I don't know . . . that adversarial, strategic kind of mind. I'm good at other stuff, but not that."

The Curious Adventurer: "Kids are always an adventure, and so is learning. I loved to read and learn about cool new stuff when I was in school. I want to help some disadvantaged kid today get that same feeling."

The Executive Manager: "When my mom or dad is preparing for a case, they're working all kinds of crazy, unpredictable hours. I like the academic calendar. The semester start this day, ends that day, classes start and end every day at the same time, and you have Christmas here and spring recess there. It's very structured and predictable. I like that."

The Creative: "Good teaching is all about coming up with creative ways to motivate your students. I've already got ideas for cool lesson plans that I could use if I get the chance."

The Standard Setter: "I love my mom, and I want her to be proud of me. But I don't feel like I need to be a lawyer to be successful. The world needs good teachers, and I believe I can be a good teacher."

The Meaning Maker: "I can make a bigger difference by getting a kid turned on to a great novel than by settling some corporate lawsuit. Watching some kid get turned on to a subject or just enjoying learning because I helped get them there . . . How awesome would that be?"

At a few points during Jason's Roll Call, his mom wanted to offer a rejoinder. "But . . . ," she started to say several times.

Coach Meg reminded her that she needed to listen and not impose her views. "You have to honor these voices and their needs," Coach Meg said, "even if you don't always agree with what they're telling you."

At the end of the Roll Call, Elizabeth was given the opportunity to speak. She paused a minute as she reflected on what she had heard. "Wow," she said. "By the time I heard Jason's Meaning Maker, I realized how much this idea of becoming a teacher really matters to him."

Coach Meg nodded. "Yup," she said. "This Roll Call is almost unanimous."

Elizabeth realized then that while she and her husband could play a role, they could not be the authors of Jason's life. This was his journey, and at least at the present time, he seemed pretty clear about its direction. Forcing the issue would backfire.

"You couldn't argue against his needs," Coach Meg says.

"And I think it was a very powerful experience for Jason's mom, as well as for Jason himself, to hear those needs articulated, and articulated clearly."

Jason continued on his track as an education major. By his senior year, he was student teaching in an inner-city school in Massachusetts, where, he told Coach Meg in an e-mail, there were possibilities of employment after graduation. "I think I can make a real difference here," he wrote.

That, Coach Meg thought as she read the e-mail, *is the voice of Confidence.*

DR. EDDIE: Pearl, age eighty-seven

I met Pearl, a spirited retired school principal, when I was asked to evaluate her upon my visit to a local nursing home. Pearl lived independently in her own home, and she reported falling outside, on a broken stretch of sidewalk. She was helped to her feet by a neighbor. Luckily, she didn't break any bones, although she was a bit scraped up. All she left on the sidewalk was a bit of blood—and her confidence and self-esteem.

"It was humiliating," Pearl told me when we met. "I was lying there on the ground, in front of my own home, unable to get back on my feet until my neighbor came to help me."

Pearl was lucky there were no serious injuries. But once she got back up, she no longer trusted herself on her own two feet. "After that, I just stopped going out," she admitted. She expressed amazement at how quickly she began to weaken from the lack of movement. (I was not surprised at all; I know from sad experience with older adults how quickly deconditioning can take place. That "use it or lose it" advice? It seems to apply doubly when you're older.)

Like so many others in the downward spiral toward immobility, Pearl tried to compensate. "At first I walked around the house, holding on to the furniture so that I wouldn't fall," she told me. "After a few days even that became difficult, and I was too winded to climb the stairs to my bedroom." She couldn't even meet my eyes when she told me what had forced her into the nursing home. "I was unable to get myself off the toilet," she said with palpable embarrassment. Luckily, she had a cell phone nearby so she could call her neighbor. But imagine the ignominy of having to be rescued from your own toilet.

I felt bad for Pearl, but before I examined her, I had a feeling about what I would find.

Nothing. Or at least nothing that couldn't have been prevented.

Indeed, my physical examination of Pearl revealed no injuries, other than some healing abrasions, and only deconditioned muscles. The gaping wound I found was psychological: an acute case of "fear of falling." In the medical literature, fear of falling is the closest diagnosis there is to a crisis of confidence. Yes, Confidence—the subpersonality you've been reading about in this chapter. The problem with fear of falling arises not from the fall but from the fear. By not continuing to walk to keep her muscles strong and her sense of balance intact, Pearl became weaker and more unstable. Her fear became a reality when she started to stumble even within her home.

From a physiological perspective, Pearl's rehabilitation was straightforward. The physical therapist helped her to her feet the first day with a walker and a waist belt for safety and support. Within a couple of days, Pearl became strong enough to pull herself to a standing positon and then to move around without the walker. Pearl dutifully listened to her physical therapist and performed her prescribed movements and exercises. As her function improved, Pearl's self-esteem was restored. During my next visit, she smiled and told me, "I feel so much better about myself now." In other words, she could get herself off the toilet without assistance. Who wouldn't she feel better about that?

During the weeks of rehabilitation at the nursing home, Pearl was challenged each day to walk a little farther and increase her weight lifting. Indeed, for anyone at any age, even centenarians, resistance exercises, such as lifting light weights or getting in and out of a chair repeatedly, lead to stronger muscles. Pearl's physical therapist also worked on improving her balance by asking her to walk on foam rubber and to try standing on one leg, something seemingly rather basic that Pearl had never done before. (Have you? It's an easy way to improve balance!)

Despite her progress, Pearl was afraid to return home.

This, I suspected, was because of a disagreement within. I'd seen this before. Older adults in her position often simply give up. "I'm too old for this," they say after a session or two of physical therapy. "I can't do it. . . . It's too late." The truth is, it's not. Pearl reaffirmed it.

So the physical therapist came up with a brilliant idea. She took Pearl out for a walk on a broken sidewalk near the rehab center, a spot that was very similar the one that had caused her to fall outside her home. Like the proverbial thrown rider climbing back on the horse, Pearl gamely took on the block-long challenge.

During my last visit, I sensed a different Pearl. She proclaimed herself ready to return home. Of course, I was delighted to hear this. Our goal is always to restore independence, if possible. But I had to ask if she was certain.

"I certainly am, Doctor," she said, sitting up straight and looking me right in the eyes. "I feel stronger than I have in years."

That was a testament to a good physical therapist. But something else was at play here. All along, from the time of her fall to her triumphant return home, Pearl had been engaged in a spirited inner dialogue with the various parts of her personality, particularly her Standard Setter and Confidence. Her success in her therapy was as much a part of her managing her emotions as it was learning to balance on that foam rubber. Indeed, without the former, the latter would not have occurred.

Pearl's Standard Setter was probably telling her that she would never be able to live on her own again—and it used the toilet seat incident to prove that point. But luckily, Pearl's voice of Confidence spoke up and probably reminded her that in the past she had set her standards high. After all, had she not lived for decades on her own, independently, before the fall? I suspect also that a strong voice of Autonomy joined in the internal debate, which concluded with Pearl making the decision (one unlike that of many others in a similar situation) to put forth a serious effort in physical therapy.

Confidence comes from challenging yourself with progressively more difficult tasks and rising to the occasion. Just like all the voices, the Standard Setter needs to be heard. Indeed, after the fall, when Pearl lowered her standards, she was listening. Once her standards were raised, she rose to the occasion. This is a key point to understand about this subpersonality. It is not fixed, immutable. The Standard Setter can be reset, just as confidence can be built (or, in Pearl's case, rebuilt). Because it is low one day does not mean that it can't be bolstered the next. So be confident and don't be afraid to set your standards high!

THE CURIOUS ADVENTURER

Curiosity is an everlasting flame that burns in everyone's mind. It makes me get out of bed in the morning and wonder what surprises life will throw at me that day. Curiosity is such a powerful force. Without it, we wouldn't be who we are today. When I was younger, I wondered, "Why is the sky blue?" "Why do the stars twinkle?" "Why am I me?" and I still do. I had so many questions, and America is the place where I want to find my answers. Curiosity is the passion that drives us through our everyday lives. We have become explorers and scientists with our need to ask questions and to wonder. Sure, there are many risk and dangers, but despite that, we still continue to wonder and dream and create and hope. We have discovered so much about the world, but still so little. We will never know everything there is to know, but with our burning curiosity, we have learned so much.

That's an essay by Clara Ma, who was twelve years old when she wrote it in 2008. She entered it in a nationwide contest sponsored by NASA to name its Mars Science Laboratory rover. Clara, who lives in Kansas, entitled her powerful essay "Curiosity." Perhaps not surprisingly, given her eloquent words on the powerful human need to know, it won first place.

Nearly four years later, on August 6, 2012, NASA landed its Mars Science Laboratory rover *Curiosity*, bearing Clara's signature (it was signed on the inside with a marker in a ceremony held prior to the spacecraft's launch), on the surface of Mars. The rover's mission is charged with answering a question that has long been on the minds of people on Earth: "Could Mars have once harbored life?"

It is the curiosity behind that question and others that has driven *Curiosity*'s mission, which is still ongoing. Indeed, that is what has driven space flight since the technology became available to do it. How fitting that this rover's name makes plain the powerful human motivation behind it.

As with our other subpersonalities, the need to explore and to seek out new experiences and an attraction to the novel and the unusual are a part of our makeup. This is the part of you that is willing to take a risk, that likes new things.

While its breadth and depth vary widely, all of us have the trait of curiosity, and we may or may not act on it some of the time or all the time. Some approach the world with wonder, a sense of curiosity, and a desire to fill their lives constantly with new experiences. Others are more cautious or content with the status quo. For most, curiosity is variable, contingent on preferences and interests (some can't wait to learn the score of the football game or who won an Academy Award). You can be curious about everything or just a few things. You may not be interested in what's happening in Afghanistan, but you may be intensely curious about your best friend's new love interest.

The Curious Adventurer itself is interesting. When things are not going well and you feel down, curiosity is often what pulls you out of your case of the blues, by asking questions:

"I wonder how we can get out of this funk?"

"What would be another way to look at this situation?"

"Is there a lesson to learn or a new direction that presents itself here?"

The Curious Adventurer loves learning, loves changes. Humans have an appetite for life; we're aroused by novelty. We're not alone. Some say that novelty seeking is one of the oldest drives in life-forms, after the Body Regulator's drive for safety and balance. It is how primitive life expanded beyond its stable environment. Does no curiosity mean no life beyond basic organisms? Maybe!

Cats, of course, are notoriously curious. But other creatures may be, as well. In his 2000 book, *Wild Minds: What Animals Really Think,* evolutionary biologist Marc D. Hauser offers some fascinating examples of other animal behavior that might be described as curiosity:

- *When a common laboratory rat is placed in a maze, it immediately begins to explore. . . . With exploration comes detailed knowledge of the turf, an understanding of which way to go for food and which way to go for the exit. Curiosity allows the rat to create a road map, a directory of spatial coordinates.*

- *In many species of schooling fish, individuals leave the safety of their group to swim by and inspect the behavior of a nearby predator. Rather than wait for the predator's*

> *attack, such bold inspectors gain information that can be used to decide whether to stay or flee.*
> * *Whenever you take a dog out on a walk, even on a route that it has taken on every outing, the dog sniffs the ground, trees, and fire hydrants. . . . Sniffing allows [dogs] to extract scents that other animals have left behind. And of course, they always sign off with their own unmistakable signature.*

While Hauser cautions us not to read too much into animal behaviors, lest we ascribe to animals human characteristics. He does point out that animals are active "informavores, digesting and storing relevant information in the service of guiding behavior."

That's one definition of *curiosity*.

With humans, the trait of curiosity is broader and more complex. Curiosity is not just about seeking what's needed for survival. On the other hand, it doesn't have to be behind as ambitious a project as exploring the planets of the solar system, either. This inner voice can be the one that simply wants a new hairstyle. Or wants to try the new restaurant that opened in town, or to check out the new TV series everyone is talking about.

Those with a powerful Curious Adventurer are commonly found among the ranks of entrepreneurs. People who "reinvent" themselves, creating new lives or careers or situations, are animated by this subpersonality. "If you want to know who's most likely to be an entrepreneur, don't go to a business school and see who has taken entrepreneurship courses," said Old Dominion University professor James V. Koch in an interview that appeared in the 2013 article "Are Entrepreneurs Born or Made?" in

Entrepreneur magazine. "The more important thing is to look at someone's personality and ability to bear risks. I would stress that I'm not saying genetics is the whole thing—I do think experience and knowledge and observation and environment count. But I'm not sure you can teach somebody to love to take risks. It seems hardwired in the individual."

In a 2013 Time.com essay entitled "The Happiness of Pursuit," science and technology writer Jeffrey Kluger suggests that Americans today are inheritors of a tradition—genetic and cultural—of risk taking, one that goes back to the taming of the continent, what was then a wilderness. "[P]ilgrims to the New World were a self-selected group," Kluger writes. "Not every person suffering under the whip of tyranny or the crush of poverty had the temperamental wherewithal to pick up, pack up and travel to the other side of the globe and start over. Those who did were looking for something—pursuing something—and happiness is as good a way of defining that goal as any. Once that migrant population started raising babies on a new continent, the odds were that the same questing spirit would be bred into or at least taught to the new generations, as well."

It's a fascinating point. Think about those millions of immigrants who arrived at Ellis Island in the nineteenth and early twentieth century. Think about what it took for them to leave everything behind and risk what little they had in a country that was, for all practical purposes, completely unknown and alien to them. *They* were risk takers. Many of us are their descendants, and many newer immigrants—who have often taken similar risks—are driven by the same sense of adventure, the same curiosity, and the same willingness to gamble on a new life.

Of course, we're not saying Americans are the only curious, adventure-seeking people in the world. Far from it. Nor are they the only ones to chafe under regulations that restrict the drive to seek out the new. When proponents of democracy talk about the need for all countries and all peoples to be free, high on those lists of liberties is the freedom to exercise one's curiosity and follow it where it leads.

CURIOUS FROM THE CRADLE

Psychologist and curiosity expert Todd Kashdan offers many insights into curiosity over the lifespan. We are born curious. Think about the infant in its cradle, reaching out to the little mobile his or her parents have hung overhead. Think about the baby on all fours or in the toddler stage, exploring the house. (We childproof things because of young children's curiosity!) Children seek the new and the novel; theirs is a world of discovery and wonderment.

And then come the rules.

Do this. Do that. Stay away from there. Don't cross that line. Do what you're told, and don't ask questions. Memorize this. Memorize that. Avoid controversy. Know the limits.

This is not to say that rules aren't important. They are. Kids need to know their boundaries. But so often, rules create a structure around children that impedes curiosity and dampens their ability to explore and discover. Good schools, good parents, good educators do their best to keep the flame of curiosity burning without burning the house down.

In addition to the rules are the fears. Some justified, others inflated. The parents of the millennial generation are often accused of attempting to engineer risk out of their children's lives, cocooning their children in car seats and bike helmets and the like. Whether or not that's true, it doesn't stop new risks from arising, whether it is social media bullies or the overuse of prescription painkillers.

Older adults are also thought to be risk averse, and sometimes for good reason. They are urged to be careful about their finances and about their health; they are sensibly cautioned about falls or about falling for telephone and Internet scams. Many heed these warnings. Yet those older adults who start second careers or become adventurous travelers or triathletes are generally lauded for their boldness.

Regardless of age, we are becoming a society that sends a double message about risk: for example, we encourage and laud entrepreneurial risk taking but discourage it in other theaters of life.

What we can do, what we should do, is to encourage curiosity—our children's and our own. "Curiosity is something that can be nurtured and developed," Kashdan explains in his 2009 book *Curious?*. "With practice, we can harness the power of curiosity to transform everyday tasks into interesting and enjoyable experiences. We can also use curiosity to intentionally create wonder, intrigue and play out of almost any situation or interaction we encounter. It all starts," he says, "with wanting to know more."

Putting curiosity in the context of the Inner Family—and keeping in mind the focus of this book, which is about learning how to better manage our emotions by meeting our needs in order to thrive—what more do we need to know about the Curious Adventurer? Well, we need to understand that this voice is at the heart of any personal change. "Coaching is about igniting curiosity," says Coach Meg. "We coaches are always asking questions, like 'What would happen if . . . ?' 'What would this look like?'

When I'm with a client, I often imagine myself being the curious owl with the cocked head."

The difference is that the owl, curiously looking over its surroundings, appears comfortable perched on its branch in the forest. Making changes, however, even in the service of curiosity, usually takes us out of our comfort zone. "Step one in any change is curiosity," says Coach Meg. "Step two is taking action, which often makes you uncomfortable."

If you're stuck in a rut, wondering why you can't make changes in your life, perhaps one explanation is that the voice of your Curious Adventurer is not getting enough attention. Perhaps it is being shouted down by the Body Regulator, who, as we have seen, is generally content with the status quo and is less likely to welcome the idea of venturing outside its established routines and boundaries.

Should that be the case with you, take heart. "Curiosity is the most malleable personality trait," says Kashdan. "It can be improved."

Indeed, it can, and we'll show you how. It's time for your Curious Adventurer to set sail, to explore new horizons, which could be as distant as a new career and life or as close as the movie theater or a clothing boutique. Let's see how healthy your Curious Adventurer is and what we can do to set it on its way toward new and exciting changes. Time for our four questions.

1. What role does the Curious Adventurer play in my life, and how has it shaped me?

Your Curious Adventurer is what gets you off the couch, gets you to go out and meet new people, and gets you to try new foods. It makes life an adventure. It enjoys the unpredictable, the uncertain. It is a big source of excitement. This part of us gets excited, like the kid who can't wait to wake up on Christmas morning. What Coach Meg calls "stuckness" can result from a lack of curiosity.

"Stuckness," she says, "is usually a sign that you have two or more inner voices with opposing views. It's an ambivalent, mixed-feeling state. You want to do something, but you don't want to do it. The pros and cons, in your mind at least, are evenly matched."

If you find yourself stuck, you can tip the balance one way or the other by getting curious about what's behind the ambivalence and about what would get you unglued.

2. What story best captures the Curious Adventurer's biggest contribution to my life?

Again, this doesn't have to be dramatic and far-reaching. The contribution—the net effect—of your curiosity is simply doing something new. It could be wearing a different piece of clothing, putting a scarf on in a different way one morning, wearing a jacket instead of your habitual sweater, or changing your hairstyle.

That story could also start with you finding yourself in a negative situation. Consider the following story, which Coach Meg helped one of her clients develop. Oliver was a college professor who had been teaching English lit classes for decades and felt thoroughly stuck. He wasn't yet in a financial position to retire. Leaving his tenured job, with its summers off, excellent health benefits, and a decent salary, made no sense. Coach Meg helped Oliver craft a new story. It started with a recognition of the many benefits and positives of his academic life: the positive impact he'd had on students, the opportunities he'd enjoyed to travel to conferences and to write articles, the sabbatical that had enabled him to write a book. She also asked Oliver to engage his Curious Adventurer in areas other than Elizabethan poetry, his academic specialty. "We suggested that he pose to himself some of those what-if questions that we know often spark curiosity," Coach Meg said. "In his case, the questions were, 'What would it be like to develop a new approach in the classroom? What would it be like to teach a new class?'"

This got Oliver, well . . . curious. That summer he took a tutorial on how to set up an online class, and then, for the first time in his career, he taught a class—his survey class of British literature from Anglo-Saxon times through the era of John Milton—via computer. He also spoke with his chairperson about his "stuckness" in the classroom. She told him they needed someone to teach a section of the college's required public speaking class that fall. Because Oliver had a reputation for being a dynamic presence in the classroom, the chairperson asked whether he'd be interested in teaching it. Normally, he would have said no to such a request—particularly on such short notice. But having now opened himself up to the possibility of change and to the voice of the Curious Adventurer, Oliver asked himself the question "What would it be like to teach a class on a topic that had nothing to do with literature or poetry?" He decided it would be challenging, refreshing, and interesting. His Curious Adventurer reawakened, he returned to the classroom with renewed vigor and interest. His might be the first public speaking class in the history of his college in which students had the option to recite soliloquies from Shakespeare plays as one of their required speeches—getting extra credit for showing up in costume, no less—and it was a big hit. More importantly, Oliver's reawakened Curious Adventurer gave him a new sense of purpose in his job.

That is the professor's story. What's yours?

CRANK UP THE GEARS OF
THE CURIOUS ADVENTURER

Some people are dying to know the latest celebrity gossip; others, the latest football scores; others, the latest galaxy discerned by the most powerful telescopes. It doesn't really matter what you're curious about. More important is that you're not suppressing your Curious Adventurer, a powerful and important subpersonality. Here's how to crank up its gears:

Step 1: Ask

Here are questions to ask yourself that can help kick-start your curiosity. The answers to these questions are open ended, and the subject matter can be anything from the trivial to the profound. The key thing is to ask. If you do, you will find yourself curious about the answer to at least one of these questions:

- "I wonder what would happen if . . ."
- "What's new about this moment?"
- "What more could I learn about . . . ?"
- "What different perspective could I take on this situation?"
- "What is a new way in which could I try to . . . ?"
- "What new experience can I have today?"
- "What new possibility is there for me when it comes to . . . ?"

Step 2: Try

Once you've got the answers, try taking one new "action step" each day. This doesn't necessarily mean you have to register for a college class, visit a museum, or resolve to read *War and Peace*. This could simply be trying something new for breakfast, taking a new route to work, donning a new outfit, even using a new coffee mug.

The smallest steps off your beaten path can awaken curiosity. And remember that curiosity is contagious: The new mug might lead to a new brand of coffee, which could lead you to decide you want to grind your own beans. The new route to work could reveal a new restaurant you weren't aware of or a new park to explore, which could in turn lead you to a nature walk on which you begin to discover the wonders of the natural world around you.

Where exactly these new steps take you is not quite as important as the fact that you're willing to take the journey, ensuring that the vibrant voice of the Curious Adventurer is part of your internal dialogue.

3. On a scale of 1–10, how well are the Curious Adventurer's needs being met today, and how important are those needs to my well-being?

If you want to make real and lasting changes in your life—if you want to thrive—your scores in this area need to be high: 7 or higher.

Coach Meg believes a little novelty every day, or at least every week, is life giving. "A small change opens up the possibility of another small change," she says. "Many small changes lead to real, transformational change." Most people who are successful at making major changes—losing weight, changing careers, making a major move—started with incremental changes.

Even seemingly insignificant, superficial changes can help get us "unstuck." Start a conversation with a new question; move the furniture around to create a new layout; cook from a recipe you haven't tried. On a daily basis, try doing something you've not done before. By the way, picking up this book is such a step.

Keep taking these small steps of self-transformation, and you'll end up with big changes and a vibrant Curious Adventurer.

4. What can I do to better meet the needs of the Curious Adventurer?

Are you seeking enough adventure or new experiences in your life? Again, we're not saying you need to plan a trip to a rain forest, learn to pilot a plane, or change careers. As mentioned earlier, what people choose to do to ramp up their curiosity quotient is often quite modest—and sometimes it can even please that risk-averse Body Regulator. "I've had coaching sessions where someone's Body Regulator says it's not okay to change careers or even to disrupt the evening schedule by taking a class," Coach Meg says. "But it's okay to take public transportation to work once in a while, instead of the car. If that's all the change you're comfortable with right now, that's okay."

In fact, it might be preferable. If your confidence level is low, even if the voice of your Curious Adventurer is robust, taking on a big change when you haven't thought it out can erode your confidence further. A brand-new runner may say, "I wonder what it would be like to run the Boston Marathon?" That's fine. It's healthy curiosity, and it's nice to dream big. But if running Boston becomes the goal before you can run even a mile, it could be counterproductive. It's a long way from going around the block to running 26.2 miles. It could lead to frustration, procrastination. It could cause your big, transformative change—becoming a runner, losing weight, getting fitter—to stall. Perhaps a better way for the curious Boston Marathon aspirant to frame that topic would be to ask questions related to the beginning and intermediary steps in that process, such as:

"What would it take for me to become a regular runner?"
"What kind of training would I have to do?"
"Once I've gotten to the point where I can run five or ten miles, I wonder what it would take to move up to the marathon level?"

Small, measurable, incremental steps. That's the way to fan the flames of curiosity and make change. Here are some other tips on how to ignite the Curious Adventurer.

Create experiments rather than commitments

Viewing your action steps as experiments takes the pressure off the Standard Setter. By doing that, your curiosity-driven actions need not be viewed as succeed/fail propositions, which would provoke an inner critic to say, "You need to get it done, or you're a loser." By saying that the action step is an experiment, and that you don't know if it's going to work, but you're going to find out, you've reframed it. Now it's simply an investigation, a fact-finding mission. Not a test of your self-worth, your ability, or your competency.

Get curious about others

We're not talking about the private lives of Hollywood stars, but if that's what helps get your Curious Adventurer's boat afloat, fine. What we're suggesting here is that you help fan the flames of curiosity by getting more interested in what's going on in the lives of those around you. Maybe you're not curious enough about your spouse or partner's day. You are concerned only about whether it went well or not, and if it did not, you wonder how that's going to affect his or her mood at the end of the day. Or when it comes to your aging parents, are you really curious about how they feel, how they are getting along in their lives, or are you mainly concerned about whether they can still live on their own? Yes, one way you can produce more curiosity within yourself is to focus on the lives of those you care about. They'll appreciate it, too!

Fall in love with change

"My genetic makeup is wired as an entrepreneur to need change," says Coach Meg. "Which is why I changed my career at age forty-two and started over in a whole new field, moved to a new country, *and* got married." Not everybody wants or needs such extreme disruptions. But change in some area or another is inevitable. The reality is that the world is always changing. The Curious Adventurer is in sync with nature, which is always changing, like the seasons, like the weather.

The Greek philosopher Heracleitus is often credited with the most famous saying about change. The original versions goes, "Ever-newer waters flow on those who step into the same rivers," and it is generally paraphrased as "You can't step into the same river twice."

Like the flowing waters, the world is constantly changing. Use your Curious Adventurer to embrace it—gradually, even, and in small ways.

Stay curious when things go wrong

"I have not failed," said Thomas Edison. "I've just found ten thousand ways that won't work."

What can we learn from the inventor of the electric light-bulb? Plenty. Edison reminds us that when it comes to innovation and change, failure *is* an option—maybe one that should be expected. But the important thing is to learn from it and move forward.

CASE STUDIES:
The Curious Adventurer

COACH MEG: Mary, age sixty-one

Mary lived a life of comfortable routine. She had been married to the same guy for thirty-five years. Her kids were grown. She and her husband both worked and were looking toward retirement in a couple of years.

Mary's days followed a predictable pattern. She got up and made her husband's breakfast: two eggs sunny side up, rye toast, a banana, and coffee. He, too, liked his routines. She went to work. Mary was a tax accountant. For twenty years, she had worked for the same firm, just a few minutes from her home. Outside of changes in the tax codes and the introduction of new computer software (it was a scary thing when she had to learn how to e-file a couple of years back), the job had also remained fairly constant. Her clients—mostly individuals and a few small businesses—trusted her, as did her boss.

So what brought Mary to Coach Meg? "Predictability," says Coach Meg. "Mary knew that she was in a rut. And even though most aspects of her life were good, she told me she had the feeling that she was living her own version of *Groundhog Day*," the 1993 film starring Bill Murray about a man who becomes stuck in time and wakes up to the same day . . . day after day.

Mary didn't like taking risks when it came to her clients' tax deductions. Why raise red flags for the IRS? But that prudent approach in her career had spilled over to other aspects of her life, paralyzing her ability to change. After years of talking herself out of trying anything new, and muting her Curious Adventurer, Mary realized that she was stuck. Of course, when she came to see Coach Meg, she didn't realize she had a Curious Adventurer. The Inner Family system was all new to her. She was intrigued. Newness was something she clearly craved, even if it entailed a new conceptualization of herself.

Coach Meg did a Roll Call and was impressed by Mary's candor as Mary tapped into each of the nine aspects of her personality:

Autonomy: "I've been doing the same thing for so long, and so much of my effort has been aimed at being a good mother and wife, that the identity I had as a young single got set aside. I'm pretty sure that this part of me wants more fun and a more colorful life."

The Body Regulator: "Don't do anything rash here. I've got a good, safe routine that's working well. I would be up, though, for trying some new exercise. My friend Patty does Zumba, and that sounds fun. I'm stuck in a rut here as far as that's concerned, just walking the dog every day."

Confidence: "This idea of shaking everything up isn't me. Remember, the grass is always greener, as they say. I may take some risks and regret it."

The Creative: "If I'm going to change, how about getting creative? I used to like to paint when I was a kid. Why don't I do more of that?"

The Executive Manager: "This could get pretty disorganized. I might not get everything done at work or at home if I'm distracted by all this emphasis on change and new stuff."

The Relational: "What will my family think of this? I'd better check in with them. My kids might not want to see me posting on Facebook or Twitter, bungee jumping, or wearing spandex at a Zumba class. And my husband might not want to join me at the French film festival that the local arts cinema is hosting this weekend. I want to check out . . . or go to the sushi restaurant I'd like to try. He freaks out over the idea of eating raw fish."

The Curious Adventurer: "I've been asleep for a long time. It's time to wake up."

The Meaning Maker: "I'm sixty-one. I'm at a point in my life where time is starting to get important. I read in *AARP* magazine that the brain slows down if you're not challenging it with new and interesting things. I haven't done anything new since I learned Quicken! When I'm on my deathbed, will that be the biggest achievement I can point to . . . the most exciting new thing I've done? There's still time to do valuable and important things with my life. I just need to figure out what they are and get moving."

So what did Mary do to satiate her Curious Adventurer? Run off with a man who loved French films and sushi? No, what she did, with Coach Meg's encouragement, was begin to make some small but satisfying changes in her life.

First, she bought an e-reader and started downloading new

books to read. She also bought an espresso machine. She had tried espresso once after dinner at a restaurant and remembered thinking how much she liked the taste. So now she reads and sips espresso. The reading led her to the local library, which, in turn, led her to a book club whose members were women of various ages. She and one of the younger moms there talked about gyms and fitness. "Have you ever tried yoga?" the young woman asked. Mary hadn't. It turned out the other woman worked as an instructor at the local yoga studio. "We have a restorative class on Saturdays you might like."

Mary hasn't made radical changes in her life; she hasn't rushed impulsively into anything. But at age sixty-one, she's escaping from her "stuckness" and beginning to allow her innate curiosity to guide her to some interesting places in life. Oh yes, and she took the restorative yoga class, found it a little too static for her liking, but while there, she heard about a Zumba class offered at the same studio. She's now a regular in that class and loves it!

Dr. Eddie: Sarah, age thirty

Early in my clinical career, I encountered what I would previously have called a "resistant patient." Sarah was a thirty-year-old stay-at-home mother of two school-age children. She came to my office with complaints of weight gain, tiredness, and an aching hip. She acknowledged some improvement from a month of physical therapy but admitted that she was not following through on the prescribed exercise program to further her gains. Sarah was certainly not the first patient to tell me this.

"Let me guess the reason you're not exercising," I said, confident that I had heard every excuse in the book. "You can't find the time."

Sarah shrugged and sighed. "Actually," she said, "once I get the kids on the school bus, I have most of the day."

"Well," I continued, "many of my patients tell me they don't have a good place to exercise. Is that your problem?"

She shifted uneasily in her seat. "We have a family membership at the new Y. It's close to my house, and I could go there pretty easily."

This was unusual. But I still had another excuse card or two to play. "Okay, so some of us just never get into the habit of exercise. We think it's sweaty and messy and involves a lot of 'no pain, no gain'-type discomfort. Is that the problem here, Sarah?"

She smiled ruefully. "To be honest, Dr. Eddie, I was a soccer player in high school. I loved practices, and I loved being in shape."

Now I was getting exasperated. I had expected her excuse for not exercising was one of the typical ones people had.

"Okay," I said. "I give up. You say that you have the time to exercise, that you have the place to exercise, that you know that it makes you feel good. So . . . ," I paused for dramatic effect. "Why aren't you exercising?"

She drew a long breath and looked up after what seemed like an eternity. "That's a great question. I need to think about it and get you an answer."

She must have done a lot of thinking, as I didn't see Sarah for a couple of months. She finally showed up and gave me her answer. "Boredom," she said. "The physical therapy exercises were deadly boring, so I realized that I stopped because it wasn't interesting."

But she had heard some of the mothers at the bus stop talking about how much they liked the exercise classes at the Y and how much fun they were.

"I finally just went over to the Y, just to see what they were offering and what these women were talking about. I heard this loud music down the hall. It was the middle of the morning. I followed the sound and walked into an aerobics class. There was my friend Tammy! And a couple of other women from the bus stop. Tammy waved me over and said, 'Come on. Just follow along.' The music was good, so I did. It was challenging at first, and I couldn't keep up, but I decided I'd come back. The next time it got easier. I was a little sore, but it reminded me of my soccer days and all those good feelings I had back then."

Better conditioned, Sarah told me all this in one excited breath. Still, it wasn't the bus stop or the instructor or the music that had motivated her, although those were all factors. Curiosity was what had really got Sarah to start exercising. My questions had sparked her thinking. What, indeed, was keeping her from exercising? She had been curious to find the answer, and once she'd realized that it was a boredom issue, it was her Curious Adventurer that got her over to the Y.

Sarah wasn't the only one who learned something from this experience. So did I.

I was curious, as well. I wondered if my patients would be more cooperative if I stopped trying to tell them what to do. The answer, it turns out, is an unequivocal yes, and ever since I made this discovery, that's how I have approached my so-called resistant patients. They don't need lectures from me about exercise; they just need to exercise their own curiosity.

As Coach Meg notes in this chapter and elsewhere in the book, the very calling together of the Inner Family—the Roll Call—is in and of itself a curious, inquisitive process. I'm sure that whether she knew it or not, Sarah was responding to some members of her own Inner Family in her efforts to find answers—most notably, of course, to her own Curious Adventurer, but also to her Body Regulator, who reminded her about how good she had felt when she was in shape as a soccer player.

Of course, the questions don't have to be about fitness or health; they could be about career issues or relationships or anything else. But unless we get curious and do the Roll Call and ask the questions, we will remain locked in our current patterns, unaware of how the different aspects of our personality are influencing our behavior.

Years later, who should walk into my office but Sarah. I barely recognized her! She was thinner and had that good healthy glow. She said she was in the neighborhood and wanted to tell me about how her first experience with that aerobics class had ignited her fitness adventure-seeking spirit. This had led her to yoga, Zumba, and boot camp. She was now taking classes to become a certified fitness instructor.

She felt great, she looked great, and the only resistance now was the weight training she had added to her repertoire.

How does Sarah's example apply to your life? Think about it. It was curiosity that probably compelled you to pick up this book. And if you have read this far, you've already further demonstrated your curiosity, your desire to learn more about your own mind and how to listen more carefully to your inner dialogue and the different subpersonalities. Keep it up. Keep asking yourself questions! Not only about healthy habits you'd like to adopt, but about those you already have. The drive and the discipline that get you to your doctor's office every year for a checkup and the appropriate medical tests could also be harnessed to get you to exercise more regularly or to get more sleep.

While you're at it, think about Coach Meg's questions for kick-starting your Curious Adventurer, listed earlier in this chapter. Let me offer you a few more:

What would it feel like to be fit and healthy, not tired and sluggish all the time, not beating yourself up about your weight or your lack of energy or your high blood pressure? What are you curious about? How you would feel and look if you were fit and healthy, and what might happen if you exercised regularly, slept adequately, and followed a healthy diet?

If you know the answer to those questions, good for you. If you don't, pondering them might be a good way to start revving up your Curious Adventurer. Follow Coach Meg's formula—take small steps, make small changes in your physical activity, and gradually pursue diet modification. Follow Sarah's example and try an aerobics class with your friends.

Small things, big things. Commit to being a lifelong learner. Commit to listening to your Curious Adventurer.

8

THE CREATIVE AND
THE EXECUTIVE MANAGER

While our concept of an Inner Family made up of a set of primary subpersonalities is relatively new, the family itself is not.

People have probably been listening to their inner voices since time immemorial.

Not only are tensions between some of the subpersonalities common, but they're also an inherent part of having this Inner Family. Two common antagonists are the subpersonalities we call the Creative and the Executive Manager. It's not a reach to say that there are human endeavors, entire industries, built around the attributes of, and differences between, these two subpersonalities.

Case in point: The advertising business, which rests on a daily precarious balance between the "creatives" (the writers and artists who come up with the advertising messages and commercials) and the "account" side of the agency (the executives, or "suits," as they are often disparagingly referred to), which oversees the business side of the equation, deals with the clients whose products are being advertised, and makes sure that the ads are on target and delivered on time.

The hugely popular AMC cable network series *Mad Men* brilliantly portrayed the workings of a New York ad agency in what is often thought of as a golden age for advertising—the mid-1950s through the late 1960s. In addition to being a superb television drama, the series sheds light on the tension between these two groups of individuals, the creatives and the suits, and by extension, on the dynamics between two very dominant subpersonalities. In one memorable scene from *Mad Men*'s first season, creative star Don Draper (Jon Hamm) angrily tells account man and über-suit Pete Campbell (Vincent Kartheiser) to "leave the ideas to me." While the conflict between the Creative and the Executive Manager in real life may not play out as dramatically as on an episode of *Mad Men*, where careers and egos are on the line, the tension still exists, and it's one of the most common and pronounced in the Inner Family.

In some people, the Executive Manager is the stronger of the two voices. This capacity, which has been explored in neuroscience, is related to the executive functions and has long been recognized as the "CEO" of the brain. In a 2008 article entitled "What Is Executive Functioning?" for the Web site LD OnLine, clinical psychologists Joyce Cooper-Kahn and Laurie Dietzel state that "the executive functions all serve as a 'command and control' function" and help the individual "manage life tasks of all types." They offer this definition of *executive functions*: "a set of processes that all have to do with managing oneself and one's resources in order to achieve a goal. It is an umbrella term for the neurologically based skills involving mental control and self-regulation."

You can think of the Executive Manager as the "voice" of at least some of those processes that help us manage ourselves and our lives. While everyone has an Executive Manager, for some it is a more dominant part of their personality. This leads to an approach to life that is more organized, structured, and linear; where things are planned and problems thought out. But what these folks may lack is the playful and impulsive free association, spontaneity, and innovation that the Creative can spark.

Let's be careful about what constitutes the Creative. In ad agencies, as we've said, the creatives are clearly defined: they're the artists and writers who come up with the ideas for the ads. Ask people what constitutes creativity, and they'll probably mention artistic or musical ability. But Harvard University psychologist Dr. Shelley Carson, author of *Your Creative Brain,* offers a broader definition. "Creativity," she says, "is the ability to generate ideas and products that are both novel and original and useful and adaptive in some way." It's also more than the ability to create pretty pictures, as she goes on to explain. "Creativity is part of our survival mechanism as a species. It's creativity . . . our ingenuity . . . that helped us survive as a species."

The development of the wheel, the cultivation of fire—these are monumental acts of ingenuity and creativity that likely had a far greater impact on human development than cave paintings or other early forms of human artistic creativity. Carson says that while the arts are typically what most people equate with creativity (and because they can't draw or carry a tune, they incorrectly conclude they have none), there are actually several other forms. These include scientific creativity, which revolves around discovery and invention; and improvisation, which Carson calls "creativity on the fly, so that you come up with solutions almost automatically to problems that arise in your life." The latter includes artistic improvisations, such as those often associated with the live performance of jazz music. But again, improvisation is not limited to the arts. A surgeon can improvise in the middle of a procedure; a parent can improvise in their explanation or interpretation to a child to help make him or her feel better.

While those who have a Creative with a dominant voice are often good at generating ideas, they are sometimes too disorganized to get them implemented. Those who march to the beat of a loud Creative voice often never get to where they're marching, because such conventions as planning a route and making sure it's followed properly are foreign to them. (A stereotype? Not really. Carson herself wrote an article, entitled "The Unleashed Mind: Why Creative People Are Eccentric," for *Scientific American* in 2011 about the historical link between creatives and unconventional behavior.)

Again, as with the personality types made stark in the advertising world, it's not uncommon for those dominated by the Creative or the Executive Manager to distrust and even despise the other: The creative person hates structure and procedure and thinks it's boring. The person with a strong Executive Manager has disdain for the playful spontaneity associated with creativity, tends to view it as a waste of time, and regards those who are creative as dilettantes.

"I've seen this so often," Coach Meg says. "Creative people think that it's boring to be organized, that it's not cool, while those with a strong Executive Manager think that creative people are just out of control."

People who are thriving usually have a balance of both and

a respect for both—and that's where you want to get. You want to integrate all the brain's resources. Or to put it in Inner Family terms, you want the best of what every member has to offer.

It only makes sense. The demands of our times make it imperative that we listen to both. We have to be thinking creatively to respond to (and perhaps help initiate) the changes that are sweeping across society. On the other hand, if we're not organized, if we can't stay focused in this age of distraction, we're never going to get anything accomplished.

If you're someone whose Creative is dominant, but you don't listen to your Executive Manager, chances are you're late for things, you're disorganized, and your Executive Manager is upset over that. Remember, whether we think it's our strong suit or not, we all have this subpersonality. Inside even the most creative person is an Executive Manager who wants to make sure there is gas in the car, the kids get to school, the bills are paid on time, and the keys are in places where they can be found. When you let the Executive Manager manage, you get more done, you're more productive, and you can better juggle varied responsibilities. While it's not usually a punitive voice, like the Standard Setter can be, it is all about business. Coach Meg often describes the Executive Manager as "the serious one in the family."

Conversely, the serious, all-business Executive Manager needs the Creative, which is the subpersonality that helps generate new ideas, that enables us to arrive at ingenious solutions in our personal lives and on the job—no matter whether the job itself would be described as "creative" or not. It's also the subpersonality that helps us avoid getting bored and stagnant. No Creative is synonymous with less innovation, little growth, and fewer healthy changes in your life.

If you're saying, "Wait a minute. I'm not creative. I can't draw a stick figure. I'm not even good at furnishing a room," let us reassure you. Creativity is not about artistic talent. It's about taking a novel or inventive approach to any aspect of life.

If, on the other hand, you're saying, "I hate all that tedious organization-type stuff," consider this: Allowing your Executive Manager to do its job does not mean you have to become a "neat freak" or transform yourself into a dull, gray organization man or woman. Every creative idea requires execution and implementation. And your big idea, no matter how creative, will never get off your personal drawing board if you forget to show up for the meeting in which you are going to pitch it.

So you need both. The Creative provides novel and interesting ideas. The Executive Manager does the evaluation, polishing, execution, and implementation. The more we listen to the one we're not prone to listening to, the better.

Of course, that might be easier said than done. The relationship between these two parts of your personality is often complex and conflicting. The Executive Manager is afraid of the Creative, afraid of the chaos and disruption. The Creative is suspicious of the Executive Manager because it's confining and conforming.

To flourish, they have to get along. Sometimes it's a bit of a shotgun wedding, as is the case in the advertising world, where the distrust between the creative and account sides of the business continues to this day, long after the era depicted in *Mad Men*. And it will continue for the simple reason that both sides know they need each other in order to be successful.

At the very least, they need to be friends in order for you to flourish. Let's get your Creative and your Executive Manager on speaking terms.

1. What roles do the Creative and the Executive Manager play in my life, and how have they shaped me?

Look back at your life since you left school and assess the role these two subpersonalities have played. Here's how it might look.

Your Executive Manager got you in the right clothes for the job interview, got you prepared so you knew what to say, got you the job. It helped you find that first apartment, figure out your weekly budget, and keep your credit card balance from going over the limit. Essentially, it was your Executive Manager who made you executive material: it got you into the adult world as a responsible person.

But it's your Creative that has had the cool new ideas that have propelled you forward in your career. Maybe it's the part that got you hired at your company, because you had new ideas on how to do things. It's your Creative that figured out the layout of your apartment so that it looks really hip. The Creative also helped come up with the theme for the cool party you threw for your friends. It provides the spice in life. It comes up with new ideas, seemingly out of nowhere.

If none of this sounds like you, you've locked up the Creative! Let it out of its cage.

Conversely, if you got the job despite being late for the interview, and you're bursting with new ideas on the job, but only when you're able to get to work on time, then it's time to let the Executive Manager out of captivity so that you're not known just for good ideas, but also for getting those good ideas implemented.

2. What story best captures the Creative's and the Executive Manager's biggest contributions to my life?

If you're dominant in one or the other, you can come up with a story in which your creativity or organizational skills helped you. But take a little extra time to think about it, and chances are, you will find an example of when they both helped.

It might go something like this: You had to put together a presentation for a new idea you had. New ideas are your strength! Organization isn't. But this time, because the deadlines were so tight and the client was so important, you didn't fool around. You allowed your Executive Manager to get in on the action. For once, you sat down and planned it out: when you needed to get the PowerPoint done, who had to sign off on it, how you were going to schedule this in with your other work. It took just a few minutes of focus, and it helped. You got the presentation done without a huge amount of drama (and, of course, creating it was the easy part). You didn't have to stay up all night and get it done last minute. You felt in control, instead of panicking and flying by the seat of your pants.

And it was a success . . . thanks to the teamwork of your Creative and your Executive Manager.

On the flip side, you have to put together a quarterly report, and it's something you're very comfortable doing. Structure and meticulousness are your forte. You pride yourself on getting things done in an orderly fashion. But this time, along with including rows of neat numbers and concise summaries, try dressing up the report. Instead of using a plain white cover, search Google Images and find an interesting picture that conveys the essence of what you say in the report. For example, do a search of "birds soaring in the sky," find an image of an eagle or a flock of birds ascending in the air, and use that as the cover for a report showing that sales or profits or market share is up.

Or, if sales have tanked, go with a picture of the *Hindenburg*. (Just kidding about that!)

Seriously, you can even experiment with different typefaces or page layouts—nothing that would make your report difficult to read, but something that might give it (and your Creative) a little flourish.

3. On a scale of 1–10, how well are the Creative's and the Executive Manager's needs being met today, and how important are those needs to my well-being?

You might just ask the question here, "Which one of the two is dominant?" Dominant would be a score of 6 or higher. If your scores are high for both, hurrah! You've got a good balance! It's sort of ordered chaos, or chaotic order, depending on whether you lean toward your Creative or your Executive Manager.

4. What can I do to better meet the needs of the Creative and the Executive Manager?

The Executive Manager brings more structuring, more prioritizing, decluttering, putting things in alphabetical order, simplifying.

The Creative loves it when your Executive Manager lets go of structure, gets out, and gets into something new. This translates into not having a plan or goals; being impulsive, spontaneous, or improvisational; and doing things because you feel like doing them now.

How do we nurture each side?

If you're creative, here's a good way to let your Executive Manager help you. Schedule thirty minutes each day (you can break it into three ten-minute sessions, if that's convenient) for organizational tasks. Check and return e-mails, review appointments, and think about the steps that need to be taken to finish your next creative project.

If, on the other hand, you're an Executive Manager–dominated person who needs to loosen the reins on your Creative, use that half hour to get away from the computer and out of the office. Go for a walk! A walk accomplishes a lot: it's good physical activity, of course, but it's also time when you can let your mind wander, which is what tends to spark creative thinking.

By the way, a famous walker was Charles Dickens. He was known for taking long sojourns by foot at night, which no doubt is when he got some of his ideas. But as the intricate plots of his classic novels and the sheer volume of his writing suggest, he was also extremely organized and disciplined.

Henry David Thoreau was another creative rambler. In a journal entry from 1851, he extols the value of movement to the creative soul: "How vain it is to sit down to write when you have not stood up to live! Methinks that the moment my legs begin to move my thoughts begin to flow—as if I had given vent to the stream at the lower end & consequently new fountains flowed into it at the upper."

So you can be both!

MANAGING CHRONIC
(AND CREATIVE) LATENESS

One of the hallmarks of the Creative-inclined mind is chronic lateness. It's understandable that when you're being so spontaneous and free spirited, you might forget a few things, like . . . the meeting with your boss or picking up your kids from soccer practice.

This is where the Executive Manager can help. Coach Meg offers these two tips for Creative chronic lateness, which, she notes, may be a sign that your commitments are beyond your personal bandwidth. You may have simply exceeded what you can carry. If so:

◆ *Trim your sails:* Write down a list of your commitments, dividing them into those that are daily, weekly, and monthly. (Maybe your spouse or partner can help.) Determine if some of these items on your list can be jettisoned, delegated, or trimmed down. In that way, try to reduce your list of regular commitments by at least 10 percent. It's better to do fewer things well then many things poorly.

◆ *Get fifteen minutes of downtime daily:* Lateness and forgetfulness may be a sign that you need some downtime to indulge your impulses, let your mind wander, and move your body, to restore calm and balance and improve brain function. Harvard Medical School mind/body expert Dr. Herbert Benson recommends ten to fifteen minutes a day of a repetitive mindful activity (deep breathing, meditation, yoga). You can do it in the morning, to start the day on a calm footing, or in late afternoon, to reboot before the evening starts.

This integration of and balance between these two seemingly opposing members of your Inner Family is the ideal. Don't throw up your hands and think that you *aren't* creative or you *can't* get organized. Those capacities are in there, waiting to express themselves. It doesn't necessarily mean you'll be a brilliant artist or a hyperefficient CEO, but you could end up realizing more of your potential and enriching your life as a result.

CASE STUDY:
The Creative and the Executive Manager

COACH MEG: Jeanine and Kevin, early thirties

Jeanine and Kevin, both in their early thirties, were engaged to be married. They were told that before they tied the knot, they should really get to understand their differences better. And there *were* differences in their personalities, as there are in many successful relationships.

Kevin worked full-time for a major insurance company in Boston, where he wrote articles for the corporate newsletter and for publications produced for customers and employees. His job paid well, but it was generally not stimulating work. What Kevin really wanted to do was write crime and espionage fiction. He devoted evenings and weekends to hammering out a novel about a private investigator who worked for an insurance company, a tough but kindhearted ex-cop who, during a routine investigation of alleged insurance fraud, uncovered a terrorist cell.

Kevin's life was almost Walter Mittyish. He dreamed about his characters, about his book, about the great crime fiction writers he admired, about how maybe someday Hollywood would make a movie based on his book, and about who would play the lead role. (It was tailor made for someone like Daniel Craig, but then Kevin wondered if he would have to set the screenplay in London.)

Kevin wrote, read, and dreamed. And Kevin really did all this in his own time. He was notoriously quirky at work. His office was a mess. He was the guy you knew you'd have to prod several times with an e-mail to get a response. His boss tolerated him because he produced stories that top management liked, but those stories would always come at a cost in terms of gray hairs and elevated blood pressure. Kevin was always scrambling to make deadlines. The production director would scream for his material, and sometimes the Web designer would call Kevin's boss, saying there was a big hole on the home page, where Kevin's story was supposed to be.

Part of the problem was that Kevin's heart was really with his own writing. But part of it was also that Kevin was a guy who was easily distracted, a guy who liked to be spontaneous, and if that meant suddenly interrupting a profile on the top-billing insurance agent in Oklahoma to jot down a plot twist for the novel he'd suddenly been inspired to write, so be it.

The Creative was a very loud voice in Kevin's Inner Family.

Jeanine, on the other hand, seemed as if she was born and bred to be a lawyer. Her intelligence, organization, and efficiency made her a natural to follow in the footsteps of her father and uncle, both successful attorneys.

Jeanine's law school experience portended a great career ahead. Her organizational skills allowed her to do more with her time than many of her classmates could do. She was always well prepared for class. Her grades consistently kept her at the top of her class. She participated in legal clinics and moot court and served as a law journal editor.

While it can't be denied that her family connections helped her get a foot in the door at a prestigious, established Boston law firm, her interview led to a quick decision, one that the firm has never regretted. She became a business defense litigator, with specialties in securities and wrongful termination suits. She proved to be a savvy negotiator. She was the go-to attorney in the office for contract interpretation. Her work was methodical and competent.

In her personal life, Jeanine was equally efficient. Despite the often long hours she put in at the firm, she managed to budget her time well enough to get in yoga and group exercise classes four days a week before work; she volunteered at a local food pantry; and you could always be sure that her Christmas card list—which she had compiled neatly in a Word document that allowed her to print out labels—was always up to date.

Jeanine had a lot of things going for her, one of which was a diligent and dominant Executive Manager in *her* Inner Family.

Kevin and Jeanine were well aware of their differences. They had been dating for two years and had lived with each other for the past year. And they both knew that they would have to make some adjustments, especially since Kevin was eager to quit his job and make a go of it as a full-time fiction writer soon after the wedding—a plan that Jeanine viewed as dubious and, like much of what her fiancé did, poorly thought out.

The differences in their personalities were manifesting themselves not only on the job. At home, Jeanine was as methodical as she was while building a case. Everything had to be planned out and carefully considered. Kevin liked to be more spontaneous, whether it was choosing furniture for the house or making social plans with friends. There had been friction there, and it was only going to intensify as the wedding date grew near.

When a coaching friend of Jeanine's told her a little about the Inner Family system and recommended Coach Meg, she shared this with Kevin. They found the concept intriguing and agreed that getting a better understanding of their inner dialogues could help them better manage the two extremes in their personalities—what they soon learned were the Creative and the Executive Manager—and make better decisions as a couple.

"They realized they had very different Inner Families and wanted my help in sorting them out," says Coach Meg. "So we did a joint Roll Call."

The couple sat in her office, and everyone listened as Jeanine's and Kevin's Inner Families sounded off. Psychologist John Mayer, whose research forms the basis of the theories used in this book, says that subpersonalities have a perspective on themselves but also on others. And so Coach Meg encouraged Jeanine and Kevin to allow their inner voices to offer observations on the other's subpersonalities. The result was different from some of the other Roll Calls you've read so far.

Autonomy

Jeanine: "I appreciate that he's comfortable with my ambitions. He knows that my career means a lot to me. He doesn't stand in my way. In fact, he encourages me."

Kevin: "I wish I could say the same thing. I don't think she respects my choice of pursuits. I know that I want to bring alive these people I've created in my head and write these exciting stories that people will like. I'm good at it, and I know I can do it. But I'm a little concerned that she doesn't respect me, because it's not that practical as a full-time job. It's a long shot that I'll make money. It's a tough business."

Jeanine was feeling validated at this point, and Kevin was getting nervous. "He didn't think she fully respected the direction in which he wanted to take his professional life," Coach Meg says. "And he didn't want to live in her pressure cooker. This was a real conflict."

The Body Regulator

Jeanine: "I'm pretty disciplined with eating and exercise. We're on top of things. But we're nervous that he's not, and that with him being home, with no structured time, it's going to get worse."

Kevin: "It's a lot of stress for me, not doing what I want to do with my life. I lie awake thinking about it at night, so I'm not sleeping well. I end up eating junk food, and I'm not exercising. It's bad."

Confidence

Jeanine: "I'm working hard, but I don't know how far up the ladder I'm going to rise at this firm."

Kevin: "I know I can write a bestseller. But I just have to get myself in a position to try."

The Curious Adventurer

Jeanine: "I'm just concerned this is too big a risk. I like to play things safe, both in my work and at home. I'm amazed that he is so willing just to take these great big flights of fancy. I mean, giving up a nice job with a big firm and good benefits . . . to write a novel? It worries me, but in one sense I

admire it. He's got a great imagination, and he's more entrepreneurial than I am."

Kevin: "I agree! I'm more adventurous. You only live once! That's
what I'm always reminding her. I don't want to spend my
whole life doing what I'm doing now."

The Relational

Jeanine: "I really do love him, even though we are very different
people. I want him to do well. I'm just worried."

Kevin: "I wouldn't want to be married to another lawyer. She's
great."

The Standard Setter

Jeanine: "I want to be a partner in that firm, like my dad and my
uncle were. I'm working as hard as I can to reach that goal."

Kevin: "I want to write like Elmore Leonard or Frederick Forsyth.
I mean, I really want to have an impact. I want to turn out
stories that people will read and buy, and that other writers
will respect."

The Executive Manager

Jeanine: "He procrastinates, and he's disorganized. It's just the
opposite of the way we are. How is he going to make a living?"

Kevin: "Yeah, we could be more organized. But good luck. Have
you talked to my Creative lately?"

The Creative

Kevin: "She's organized. But isn't there such a thing as over-
organized? She's too structured. Everything is planned and
thought out to the max. She needs to loosen up and have fun.
That's what I do. That's what drives me."

Jeanine: "You're right. I *am* too structured and rigid. I'd like to have some fun, too, but my Executive Manager runs a tight ship here."

At about this point, Coach Meg says, Jeanine and Kevin began to reach a better understanding of each other, thanks to what was expressed in the Roll Call. "They started to realize that they each had a part that was saying, 'I do like this. . . . I would like to be a little more organized or to have a little more fun.' But those parts are not getting any attention. This is something neither of them knew before they took the Roll Call."

There was still one more subpersonality to be heard from.

The Meaning Maker

Jeanine: "Being with him is going to provide a voice for my Creative, which is being stifled. I know I need that, despite the Executive Manager's reservations, and that's a good balance for me."

Kevin: "If I want to meet my goal, if I want to make a go of it as an author, on my own, I admit I need to get a little bit more structure. I have the capability to do it. I just have to listen to it more."

Success! They were able to hear each other's Inner Family and realize that their own ignored subpersonalities had underused resources. They understood that if they could tap into those, they'd have a more balanced dynamic, one that was not so one sided.

We're not going to turn a disciplined, achievement-oriented, high-functioning Executive Manager into a spontaneous Creative. Nor is Kevin likely to become a paragon of efficiency or the neatest man in the building. What Coach Meg was looking for was a little more balance for each of them—a little more spontaneity in Jeanine's life, a little more structure in Kevin's. And that is what you should be looking for in yourself.

The couple took what they had learned from their visits with Coach Meg and from the Roll Call and began to do something about their life, something small to begin with. Jeanine went the following weekend to her nail salon and got her toenails painted a bright coral color. This was much different than her usual conservative approach. Kevin noticed. "Wow," he said when she got back. "That's cool! A little life here!"

He, on the other hand, devoted two hours a week to getting household chores done. While Jeanine could make suggestions, Kevin followed his own list of things he felt he needed to do around the house. He knew he had to make sure he got them done. He started, not unpredictably, by taking over the yard work. There was enough creativity in gardening to make him feel comfortable, but scheduling the time to mow the lawn and pull the weeds every week required that he get his underused Executive Manager involved.

These are small changes, admittedly. But that's how lasting change begins. Jeanine's and Kevin's Inner Families may never become completely balanced, and their differing subpersonalities may never totally sync in this area (not unlike real families that are brought together through marriage). But Jeanine and Kevin can learn to modulate those voices and respond to them a little bit better and, in the process, make the relationship a little more harmonious as they both pursue their career goals and their lives together.

9

THE RELATIONAL

Love can make you happy," sang the American pop group Mercy in 1969, "if you find someone who cares to give a lifetime to you."

"And when I'm gone, just carry on. Don't mourn," rapped Eminem in 2005.

These are two contrasting views on relationships expressed in song: one a sweet, hippy-dippy hit by a now largely forgotten band; the other, in the words of journalist Anthony Bozza, "a clear, dead-eyed analysis of a superstar's own failings as a father and husband."

The two songs, from disparate ages and perspectives, have one thing in common: they're both about the human need to connect to others, in the case of the first song to a partner and in the case of the second to a child, but it could be a parent or even a stranger. That's what makes the Relational unique among all our subpersonalities. It's the one that's oriented toward serving the needs of others. And this is one of its essential differences when compared to the other subpersonalities. Think about some of the members of the Inner Family whom we examined in previous chapters. The Body Regulator is about what *your* body needs to function; Autonomy is about what *you* need for self-fulfillment; the Curious Adventurer is about *you* seeking new horizons and experiences.

They're all essential parts of being human, but it's all "Me, me, me."

Relational is the one member of your Inner Family that puts others first. It's the caregiver, the parent, the nurturer.

The Relational subpersonality is one that should be familiar to most people, because we are all in relationships of one sort or another. Friends, colleagues, teachers, extended family, neighbors. Your dentist, your mechanic, your personal trainer. We have relationships of one form or another with a complex web of other individuals. And while the role of some of these people in your life may be primarily to fulfill a specific need you have, you care about them, too. As the late Dr. Christopher Peterson, a leader in the new field of positive psychology, famously said, "Other people matter."

The part of us that is concerned about those others—their needs and their welfare—is our Relational capacity.

The Relational cares, and not just about your spouse, child, or BFF. It could be the person on line at Starbucks or a stranger you read about in the news. The impulse to run over and help someone who has slipped and fallen as he or she was coming out of the supermarket is the work of your Relational. What motivates you to donate money to help the survivors of an earthquake is your Relational. It's also what drives you to visit a sick friend in the hospital or an aged relative in an assisted-living facility, or simply to buy your office assistant flowers or a gift on his or her birthday.

When asked why they raise money for a cause or volunteer, people often answer, "Because it makes me feel good." Well, part of the "me" they're talking about is the Relational. And the reason it "feels good" is that they are heeding what this voice says, addressing the need of this important drive. The Relational is pure caring, without any good reason, and as such, it is more noble and selfless than the other subpersonalities, save the Meaning Maker, which we will discuss in the next chapter.

As with the other eight subpersonalities, some of us have a stronger Relational drive than others. Nurses and teachers embody the stereotype of the person driven by the Relational. And certainly most are, but so are coaches and firefighters and cops and psychologists, not to mention people whose jobs aren't in the so-called helping professions. An accountant, an auto mechanic, an advertising designer, and a hedge-fund trainer can all have a strong need to support and care for others, too.

The Relational manifests itself differently in certain situations. Hugging your dad or gently stroking the arm of a child is one way, but so is fist bumping with the members of your basketball team, or taking part in the call-and-response chants of military drill instructors and recruits as they run.

For some, the Relational is a dominant part of their personality. Serving others gives them supreme joy. You may be like that, and you probably know others who are. Most parents and caregivers heed this voice. For some, including the folks who work in those helping professions we mentioned, the need is so powerful, the voice so strong, that they build their life's work around it. On the other hand, some of us are more introverted or choose to travel a more solitary path in life.

Still, make no mistake, all humans have the Relational capacity, and all humans need mutually caring relationships to thrive.

Psychologists Deci and Ryan, whom we first met in chapter 1, believe that people's sense of connection, or relatedness—which they define as a sense of belonging and an attachment to other people—is one of the three most fundamental human needs (along with autonomy and competence). So the nurturers among us are not the only ones for whom the Relational capacity is important.

Research has shown that social relationships are a determinant of aging well. A 2012 *New York Times* story headlined "A Longer Life Is Lived with Company" reported on a University of California, San Francisco, study showing that older adults who said they felt isolated and lacked companionship had a "45 percent greater risk of dying earlier than older adults who felt more connected to others."

Interest in the importance of relationships, and of successfully establishing and nurturing them in every phase of life, has produced a rash of books on the topic over the years. Actually, "a rash" might be an understatement. Search Amazon.com for "relationship books," and 250,035 entries come up. They have titles like *The Relationship Cure, Making Your Relationships Work,* and *Relationship Rescue.* They promise, in their subtitles, *The Secret to Love That Lasts, Ten Minutes a Day to a Better Relationship,* and *The Seven Principles for Making Marriage Work.*

This is not one of those books.

We're not relationship counselors who can show you how to deal with your adolescent child, how to build a successful marriage, or even how to interact with your aging parents (although one of our case studies in this chapter does address that very topic, albeit from a different perspective).

In this book we acquaint you with nine primary sources of human needs and drives, expressed in our positive and negative emotions and thoughts, which keep up a steady chatter inside your head. What we're trying to do in order to thrive and function at our best is to help all these subpersonalities get their needs met and get along better. But as you have seen, that's complicated. Not only do we deal with the interrelationships among our varied and conflicting subpersonalities, but when we relate to another person, we must manage how our nine primary subpersonalities interact with that person's nine subpersonalities. So that's eighteen subpersonalities in a single relationship, and if you are a family with a child, there are at least twenty-seven subpersonalities in that situation!

We'd love to be able to say that awareness of this, of the fact that your spouse, partner, or friend has his or her own subpersonalities, will make relationships easier. On the contrary. It's hard enough to manage your own needs; now you've got to account for the nine needs of someone else! This is yet another reason why relationships are challenging. This is also why it helps to understand what's going on inside our heads. Knowing that your partner's Relational or Autonomy is a dominant voice, for example, can go a long way toward helping you better appreciate and understand each other and communicate.

THE RELATIONAL VS. AUTONOMY

We've talked about the inherent conflicts between some of the members of our Inner Family. For example, we have looked at how the need for safety and security espoused by the Body Regulator can often be at odds with the needs of the more adventuresome Curious Adventurer.

These conflicts bubble up from time to time, just like quarrels in a real family. As many of us know, there are sometimes two individuals in a family who always seem to be at loggerheads. They may love each other, but they are also exceedingly good at antagonizing each other. In your Inner Family, a similar dynamic can exist, and there the bickering duo would be the Relational and Autonomy. There's an inherent tension here that pervades almost every aspect of your life: You want to live life to its fullest potential and self-actualize, but you also need to make sure you have close relationships in which you help others do the same.

These two competing drives often cause problems, not just internally but also among the people around us: Maybe when you were young, your parents were concerned when you told them that your destiny was to be a tattoo artist or a professional skateboarder, and for that reason, you were dropping out of school. Or maybe you wanted to buy an SUV, but your spouse wanted a sports car. Or perhaps when you are elderly and want to stay in your home, your grown children will think you need to be in an assisted-living facility.

Sometimes, these tensions between the Relational and Autonomy can degrade into a battle between responsibility and selfishness. Think of the stories we hear about teenagers who run away from home or parents who leave or neglect their kids to pursue a quixotic dream. It is more important for them to climb Mount Everest or jet off for two weeks on a golf outing with buddies than to be with their kids.

The message here is that life is a continual balancing act between serving your own needs and meeting the needs of others. The art of living well is to do that well.

Here are some tips from Coach Meg on how to balance these two conflicting drives:

◆ Appreciate that meeting your need for autonomy is not selfish. Nor should your inherent need to meet others' needs and to give love be seen as some kind of weakness. Both needs are deeply wired and should be appreciated and validated. They are what they are, and both contribute richness to your life.

◆ Cultivate adult relationships that are mutual, meaning that they honor and serve the autonomy of both parties. Often in parental, familial, and work relationships you focus on serving others—your children, your partner, your boss—and Autonomy's needs get neglected. This is where friends and like-minded associates can help.

◆ Set a little time aside each week to make sure you're meeting both your Relational and your Autonomy needs. Once a week, do something nice and thoughtful for someone in your life. It doesn't have to be a gift or flowers; even just a kind word will do. Once a week, be a loner. Stay home by yourself and indulge in whatever intellectual passion or hobby or pastime interests you.

◆ Also on a weekly basis, check in with both of these entities of your psyche, asking, "What more do I need to do to meet both the need to march to my own drummer and the need to serve those I care about?"

Now, let's get back to the Relational capacity, and pose our four questions to help determine how well adjusted yours are.

1. What role does the Relational play in my life, and how has it shaped me?

This is an important question for two reasons. First, with this capacity, the role changes.

When you're really young and so dependent on your parents, you're concerned about making them happy. That's the main Relational thrust. You cuddle with your parents, you give them love, and you're cute and charming. That's the attachment stage—when you feel secure and cared for.

Then you branch out beyond the love of your parents and siblings and grandparents. You establish relationships with peers and teachers when you start going to school. In adolescence, the focus of your relationships is your peers. Maybe it's just the crowd you hang out with. Or maybe it's the members of your team or, when you're in college, your fraternity or sorority. As an adult, you shift your Relational focus again, this time to finding that special relationship and perhaps to building your own family. By that time you're also in full flight in your career. You may have an immense web of relationships. So your relationships get more complex, more diverse, often more intense. The relationship types and patterns vary.

The other reason this question is particularly pertinent here is that some people are more introverted than others. Some people are happier to be alone; other people seem to need others around them. If you're the former, and you think there's somehow something "wrong" with you because you're more of a loner, think again. The Inner Family concept holds that all of us have these nine aspects to our personality, but they're not all of equal strength. Autonomy might be a more potent drive in your life. Yes, the Relational voice needs to be heard like all the others, but that doesn't supersede the simple fact that some people are quite content to spend more time alone.

2. What story best captures the Relational's biggest contribution to my life?

Is Relational's biggest role in your life manifested in your marriage? Your role as a parent? Your relationship with your parents? Or close friends who have enriched your life? Or your colleagues?

Think of examples where your relationships were a "win-win," for both your Autonomy and your Relational capacities. You can choose how to balance both drives, even if you don't get to choose your parents or your children. You choose your life partner and your friends, a great opportunity to get both needs met. And you can choose how to get both needs met with your close colleagues at work.

Consider the following three people, each with a unique balance between the Relational and Autonomy. The first is happiest when serving others; he or she is the family chaplain and listens to people's problems. The second is a person who has a balanced life, one filled with family, friends, and a career. The third person is one who is a high achiever and, consequently, has less time for family and friends but has great work relationships.

Just because you have a deep need for Autonomy doesn't mean you're selfish. And just because you have a strong Relational need doesn't mean you're someone without a sense of self. These are independent elements of your personality that interact closely throughout your life. As long as you appreciate what both of these needs are, and you make sure that they're being met—and are not squelched by a louder, more domineering subpersonality—you'll be more likely to flourish.

3. On a scale of 1–10, how well are the Relational's needs being met today, and how important are those needs to my well-being?

This is going to depend. For a mom with enriching hobbies or work projects, with grown kids and grandkids who are all doing well, it's going to be a 9 or a 10. For the woman who has a rewarding career and who is unmarried but has nieces and nephews that she's close to and many close friends, it could still could be a 9 or a 10. Those relationships can be just as important.

The key question in this self-assessment is: What would enable me to thrive more? Here are four different ways to interpret the scores that may help answer that critical question:

- If the "need being met" score is low or medium and the "need is important" score is high: *"Life would improve if I invested in more relationships."*
- If both scores are moderate: *"Maybe there's no need to rock the boat."*
- If the "need being met" score is high and the "need is important" score is medium or low: *"I could divert some resources to focus on meeting other needs."*
- If the "need being met" score is high and the "need is important" score is high: *"I'm doing what I need to thrive!"*

4. What can I do to better meet the needs of the Relational?

Developing successful relationships involves listening to others and serving others. You're making time for them, you're helping them, and you're engaged and involved in their needs. As the saying goes, you are "there" for them—which is often considered the definition of a true friend.

It almost always pays to broaden your Relational scope. Those individuals whose needs you serve could be complete strangers. A strong Relational often manifests itself as giving time to volunteer organizations or making a difference through charitable giving. That good feeling you get when you've helped out at the local homeless shelter or donated money to a worthwhile charity? That's your Relational capacity smiling.

Another look at the results of that search for "relationship books" on Amazon.com reveals that the top fifty bestsellers are about relationships with members of the opposite sex. Further down in the top one hundred, a couple of titles pop up about relationships with your child or with a same-sex partner. But it's not until you nearly reach result number two hundred that a book appears about aging. And yet, as we've said, your Relational needs encompass a wide range of people and interactions. Relationships with aging parents are a conundrum for many young and middle-aged adults in particular—not to mention the parents—as our case study illustrates.

CASE STUDIES:
The Relational

COACH MEG: Florence, age seventy-six

Martin was a forty-one-year-old banker. His mom, Florence, seventy-six, was a retired elementary school principal. Florence's husband died years ago, and while she seemed to have done well living alone, she was starting to become a bit more limited physically and isolated. Martin was concerned, and he wanted her to move out of her home, where she had been living for nearly forty-five years, and into a senior-living facility.

When Martin approached his mother about this, the conversation didn't go well. He was blunt, telling her that he'd noticed that she had difficulty climbing stairs. He pointed out that she rarely seemed to leave the house anymore. "When's the last time you went to a movie with your girlfriends?" he said.

Proud of her independence and resentful of what she saw as her son's intrusion into her social life, Florence took umbrage at this. The argument continued, and after they parted ways, they didn't speak for a few weeks. Then Flo tripped and fell while she was bringing laundry up from the basement. Luckily, no bones were broken, but she had a big bruise on her arm, which Martin couldn't help but notice when he came by to make amends.

"Mom!" he said. "I'm sorry about getting on your case about this, but certainly you've gotta see now that we need to start discussing this issue of your living situation."

Reluctantly, Florence agreed, but she said she'd feel more comfortable if someone else was there, "somebody who knows what they're talking about."

After a flash of indignation over this apparent insult, Martin tried to practice the deep breathing exercise he'd learned in the lunchtime yoga class his company offered to help employees reduce their stress. It worked. He regained his calm demeanor and shrugged. "Okay, Mom. Maybe that wasn't the nicest way to say it, but you're right," he said. "I'm not an expert on this, and it's an important decision."

He told her he'd try to figure out the right person to give them advice, but as he walked out of her house that day, he realized he wasn't sure whom he should contact. An elder-care lawyer? A friend of the family? A therapist? A physician? Who would be the appropriate professional? And whose help would his mother accept? Then he recalled that his friend Nikki had worked with a coach to reengineer her life. He called her.

"Yes, of course," she said when Martin inquired as to whether she thought a coach could help in this situation. "That's kind of what they do. They help you with change, like the way I had to change to reorganize my priorities."

This was a very different kind of "change" for Martin to tackle, but he decided to approach Nikki's coach about working with his mom. Coach Meg agreed, as long as Florence was amenable to the idea.

To Martin's surprise somewhat, she was. "I like the idea of having someone coach me," Florence told Martin. "But I hope this one isn't like those football coaches on TV. They're always yelling or arguing, and they look so fierce and serious."

Martin assured her that Coach Meg did not bear the slightest resemblance to a college or NFL coach and that her work was not at all like coaching football.

When they met, Coach Meg explained the concept of multiplicity of mind—that is, the model of the nine primary subpersonalities or entities of the psyche—to Florence, who seemed to find it quite interesting. They talked a little bit about the discussions she and her son had been having, and then they did her Roll Call to get a better sense of how Florence's Inner Family was reacting to Martin's entreaties:

Autonomy: "I've been in charge of my life for all my life after age sixteen. I worked myself up the ladder of the public school system, earned a master's degree at night, and raised a family. Of course I'm capable of living by myself!"

The Body Regulator: "I have mixed emotions. If I were in a more structured place, I'd be in the gym more often. And that would be good, because while the occasional walks in the neighborhood are nice, I need a more regular routine. But I like to cook and eat my own food, so that's not so good. And I love to sleep in my own bed."

Confidence: "I am competent, and I've proved it throughout my working life. I don't want to see myself as incompetent. It's important that I'm out in the world, that I live in a community surrounded by people of all ages. I like having young families as neighbors and interacting with young people when I shop. I want to be with people who are sharp, and it's a mixed bag in these assisted-living places. I want to hang out with smart, accomplished people like me, not with a bunch of cranky old people."

The Creative: "I really don't do a lot of creative stuff at home. I don't really know where to start. I hear they have art classes at these places. Maybe I'd be more creative if I was around others engaged in creative projects."

The Curious Adventurer: "I'm free to travel, but I could use some friends who could push me to try new things. I'm kind of locked in to my routine. I'm not plugging myself into new stimuli."

The *Executive Manager:* "I'm on top of my finances. I keep up with everything. I've got a good accountant, a handyman, a lawn service. I don't need to hand this off to someone else. Besides, I like keeping my household finances, making my shopping lists, and organizing my day. I read that working memory declines when you retire, so it's good for me to be doing those things, anyway. If I don't organize my day and engage in different activities, my brain will turn into mush."

The *Relational:* "A lot of my old friends have retired and moved away. It's one thing to wave hello and exchange small talk with that young couple next door, but I need more engaged social relationships than that. I need friends who might want to take an art class with me or fly to London for a long week-end. And Autonomy needs to know that there will be a time when we *have* to sell the house. But we can still have control and make it a softer landing when we do. Friends and family will help in that transition, as well. And I agree with the Creative and the Curious Adventurer. We need more new things to do, and with different people."

The *Standard Setter:* "I want to be self-sufficient and to live on my own for as long as possible. I agree with Confidence. I think I'm strong enough to take care of myself. I want to show others how to age well, which is by staying active and sharp. I don't want to be surrounded by people who are dependent on others for everything."

The *Meaning Maker:* "I feel good, and I think I'm doing pretty well for a woman my age. But I am aging, and I have to accept the fact that at some point I will need to give up both the house and the car and move to a place where I can get a little more help. Let's be clear, though, that this is not yet the time. So I don't want to just ignore my son's comments. He's concerned, and I appreciate that. And he's right that I should begin to think about when that day comes that I can't stay here. But I want to be the one to decide that and to decide where I go and what happens to me."

After Florence's Roll Call, in which her Meaning Maker seemed to help manage the conflicts between her Relational and Autonomy, Coach Meg and Florence did a debriefing. "We talked about how she could acknowledge her son's concerns, while still asserting her own control over her life," Coach Meg says.

They discussed ways in which this could be achieved. Florence mentioned that she had a friend who lived at a nearby senior-living facility who had been asking her to come by and visit. Among other things, the friend had raved about the gym and the people who worked there. "You should come and take a dance class with me," her friend had told her.

"I've been meaning to try it," Florence said to Coach Meg. "Maybe now's the time."

While Florence said she was quite happy most nights in her comfy chair with a book in hand or the TV on, she knew that she needed to find some ways to be a little less socially isolated, which seemed to be one of Martin's concerns. Florence and Coach Meg brainstormed on how she could get more connected to interesting, smart people. She told Coach Meg about a younger colleague of hers who was still teaching. She had been a mentor to this teacher, and they were overdue for lunch together. There was also a group of retired teachers she knew, several of whom liked to walk together at a nearby mall several mornings a week. This was a social activity that could get her into a steadier exercise regimen. And there was her niece, Jessica, who lived in North Carolina and had been asking her favorite aunt to come visit and see her baby.

"Maybe it's about time I did that," Florence said to Meg. "In the winter maybe, when I'm a little more stuck in the house. And Jessica's a love. I haven't spent much time there in the past few years."

Florence was addressing a number of needs here, and while Martin's concerns had certainly helped spark this process of self-examination, it was the Relational that was now asserting itself. As the old telephone company ads used to say, she needed to "reach out and touch someone." And, in turn, be touched by a few someones. Former colleagues; friends, both older and younger; relatives. It didn't really matter who, as long as they fulfilled that human need for engaging, meaningful relationships. In this case, Florence's need for autonomy and relationships and adventure could all be met at once if she visited other people and shared daily life with them more often. In short, she had to listen to her Relational voice.

Dr. Eddie: Gino, age thirty-seven

Gino, an affable software salesman, arrived in my office one morning with an outstretched hand and a mile-wide smile. Gino had a recurring ankle sprain and had been under our care for a few months. He was just completing a course in physical therapy and had been faithfully doing his daily exercises. (I knew this not only because I had read the reports from his PT, but also because Gino himself had dropped by a few weeks earlier to inform me personally of this fact.)

"Good morning, Doc," he said cheerfully and then immediately began to apologize. "I hope I'm not wasting your time today. I just wanted to come by to tell you in person that my ankle pain is pretty much gone."

I was, of course, happy to hear about Gino's progress, but admittedly, I was a bit surprised. Gino had distinguished himself from my other patients by showing up to report that his pain was resolved. Although I routinely scheduled follow-up appointments with all my patients, truth be told, most of those who were feeling better tended to cancel their follow-up appointments. They just got on with their lives. Gino seemed to have stopped by my office for other reasons. And, to be honest, I was glad he did.

"I'm never too busy to hear some good news!" I told him as we shook hands. "I'm also happy to see you with or without pain. Tell me the secret of your success."

He chuckled. "Come on, Doc. You know the answer to that. I listened to you, and I did what the physical therapist told me to do. I mean, the exercises were a little boring, but she was great, and she seemed really pleased to see me doing them. It's just kind of too bad that . . ." Gino's voice trailed off.

"What's too bad?" I asked him.

"Well, it's just too bad that I'm getting discharged from PT just as it's starting to help me. I guess it's different from sales, where I'm always looking to get to know my customers better, always working on building these relationships. We're never 'done' or 'finished' in sales. But in your line of work, I guess, the injury heals, and then it's 'So long!'"

I couldn't help but smile at this. So often, patients can't seem to wait to get out of our office or to complete their physical therapy. And here was Gino, wishing to extend his time with us.

He was certainly a people person, and his Relational voice sang loudly. He was happy to try to build the relationship with the physical therapist (and to please her by doing the exercises). He even went out of his way to keep his appointment with me to further our relationship.

"Gino, I appreciate that," I said. "And I want to tell you that even though your ankle's doing better and you're pain free, I'd be happy to continue seeing you, to coach you along so that you get even stronger and can then resume some more regular exercise. You know, some of my patients rehab to one hundred ten percent and end up stronger and fitter than they were before their injury."

"Wow. That's cool," said Gino. "I'd love to get stronger and in better shape. It would really help my tennis game."

I'm sure it would, I thought to myself. But I knew it would also help something else that was very important to Gino: his Relational capacity, which was obviously a dominant voice in his Inner Family. *This,* I realized, was really why he was here. Upon later reflection, in the midst of my own Roll Call, I realized upon listening to my own Relational voice that I, too, was there in that exam room in part because of the relationship.

My offer to have Gino back next month to begin a general conditioning program enabled us to continue that relationship. I looked forward to seeing him.

Unfortunately, most of my patients are not quite as outgoing or as eager to spend time with me as Gino is. So many just seem to come and go. For me, and for many other physicians, the pace and stress of modern health care can be overwhelming at times. The demand to see more patients faster, while documenting these visits in ever-changing electronic record systems, can feel dehumanizing. However, as a people person myself, I try to follow the advice of my colleague Dr. Edward "Ned" Hallowell (a preeminent writer on the subject of attention-deficit/hyperactivity disorder) to utilize the connection prescription. His advice is to "make eye contact, smile, and say hello to ten people per day. It will change your mood and improve your health." I've tried it, and it works, even with strangers. On the days when I see patients, I can go well beyond the simple hello and really attempt to connect. While they may not all be like Gino, with a bit of persistence and by closely listening to their spoken and unspoken words, I've found that a connection is formed. My life is richer for that.

My experience with Gino was a reminder that even in the midst of a busy, overscheduled day, you can slow down and take the time to connect to whomever you meet by making eye contact and listening carefully to what they are saying. Even a brief connection is helpful.

Improving your health and wellness need not be a solitary activity. Remember, Gino did best when he felt connected and accountable to his caregivers. Consider joining groups or staying in touch with others as you make changes in your health behaviors, such as losing weight and getting active or whatever else you would like to change.

We are at our root social beings. Connect with those around you so that you don't feel alone.

10

THE MEANING MAKER

In May 2015 *New York Times* columnist David Brooks invited readers to submit essays describing their purpose in life and how they found it. He received thousands of responses and shared some of them in two subsequent columns. Not surprisingly, many of his readers had found their purpose in life through raising children, caregiving, or managing and influencing others.

One man—who had been given a reprieve by a sympathetic police officer after a youthful transgression—wrote that his purpose was to mentor.

A woman was using the experience she gained while navigating her way through the health-care system for her brain-injured brother to help others.

An older man said he found his day-to-day purpose in tending his garden.

The meaning of life found in tending a garden? Why not? "I expected most contributors would follow the commencement-speech clichés of our high-achieving culture: dream big; set ambitious goals; try to change the world," Brooks writes in one of those subsequent columns, "The Small, Happy Life." "In fact, a surprising number of people found their purpose by going the other way, by pursuing the small, happy life." One of the readers whose essay he quotes had this to say on the matter: "Perhaps . . . the mission [of life] is not a mission at all. . . . Everywhere there are tiny, seemingly inconsequential circumstances that, if explored, provide meaning."

In the context of the Inner Family, what Brooks and his respondents are addressing is the capacity, the subpersonality, that we call the Meaning Maker.

This ninth, most advanced subpersonality is one of the most complex. And unlike some of the other subpersonalities, which reflect needs that are shared by other life-forms, this is a distinctly human one. No other creature, as far as we can tell, recognizes its own mortality and ponders the existence of an afterlife.

As its name suggests, the Meaning Maker is the capacity within us that seeks wisdom, strives to make sense of and find purpose in our lives. It is a philosopher, a counselor, a minister and, given its role of mediating between the competing needs of the other subpersonalities, a diplomat.

It's also a strategic thinker, concerned with big picture issues.

The needs it addresses are equally complex. As opposed to the Body Regulator, which is concerned with the primary drives for food, safety, and so forth, the Meaning Maker helps us with our need for transcendence, meaning and purpose, awe and gratitude, and harmony.

Not everyone finds their purpose in life, and as Brooks's column suggests, most of us find it in different ways. It's not surprising, then, that purpose is a common issue that coaches help their clients deal with.

"Helping people make meaning of their lives is a big part of what we do," says Coach Meg. "They ask, 'What should I work on right now?' 'What's the most important change I can make in my life?' 'How does this matter?' 'How will that make me a better person or affect my legacy?' Typically, people look for a coach because they're stuck. And often what they're stuck on are the big questions."

If it sounds like the Meaning Maker is the provenance of those who attend church, read philosophical tomes, or sit and stare up at the stars, contemplating their existence, don't be mistaken. This capacity is common to all humans, not just those with an uncommon intellect. It's not a capacity that only Plato, Albert Einstein, Ayn Rand, and Martin Luther possessed and that the Dalai Lama exhibits. Although, of course, those who have devoted their life's work to making meaning no doubt have a very dominant Meaning Maker in their Inner Family. Nor is this capacity devoted solely to the big questions of existence, which these great intellects pondered.

"It's not only about 'When I die, will my soul live on?'" Coach Meg says. "It's also about 'How do I find the right answer to the problem I'm facing today?'"

Both people of faith and religious doubters have the Meaning Maker capacity.

Indeed, coming up with a graphic representation of the Meaning Maker is challenging, because it changes its shape depending on the role it's being call on to play. It could be envisioned as a professorial sort with a tweed jacket, a white-bearded old sage in a cloak, or a wise matriarch. It could be a sports official in a zebra-striped shirt, blowing a whistle. It could be the well-appointed person at a conference room table, who sits quietly as an issue is debated by the others in attendance and speaks only after the others have expressed their views.

The Meaning Maker is all these and more.

Earlier in this book, we talked about the Mindful Self. Some might wonder about the distinction between this entity and the Meaning Maker. Although no one knows for certain, it's likely that the Mindful Self doesn't have a distinct voice, unlike the nine subpersonalities. It listens to all the subpersonalities, who then work together to produce the voice that we use to speak to the world.

The Meaning Maker, however, is certainly one of the nine subpersonalities, albeit one that is more reflective and measured than the others. As opposed to the Mindful Self, the Meaning Maker can be conceived of as the higher self, which is why our discussion of it treads onto turf usually occupied by philosophers and theologians.

You'll note that in the Roll Calls included in the case studies in previous chapters, the Meaning Maker speaks last. That's deliberate. This is the capacity that takes in what the others have to say, synthesizes their needs, and often helps broker a solution.

"In situations of personal distress," says Coach Meg, "it's the one who puts the proverbial hand on our shoulder and says, 'It's going to be okay.'"

In your internal conflicts, the Meaning Maker can be a peace-keeper. It appreciates and honors the contributions of all your other subpersonalities in the inner debate. And then, if asked, it suggests a sensible course of action.

That's not to say that the Meaning Maker doesn't deal with those big questions. If you *are* a person who attends a house of worship, your Meaning Maker has probably helped you arrive at that place. If you pray or have conversations with a higher power—whether you call it God, Jesus, Allah, the Force, or something else—this is likely the part of you that channels that connection.

Discerning this voice amid those of your other subpersonalities is not easy. Unlike some of the other subpersonalities, which emit more plaintive cries in the inner dialogue—"I'm hungry" (the Body Regulator), "I'm frustrated" (Autonomy), "I'm bored" (the Curious Adventurer), "I'm lonely" (the Relational)—the Meaning Maker is more subtle, and tuning in takes time and effort. It can be difficult for younger people to hear their Meaning Maker. The Meaning Maker, like the other subpersonalities, seems to grow and develop over time. But because the other subpersonalities can be rambunctious, we often assume the loudest voice is the defining voice of our personality. So we feel an emotion and think, *That's me. That's who I am. I'm angry.* As we get older, we realize that it is but one voice of many and that these emotions will pass. The Meaning Maker helps nudge us toward that realization; it helps us to embrace the multiplicity of mind that is part of all of us.

And yet while it may be there to help us sort out some of life's ambiguities, to make our minds up when faced with complex decisions, the Meaning Maker can play a very practical role, as well. Suppose you're in a situation in which some members of your Inner Family are agitated and noisy. The Meaning Maker is the subpersonality that can help find the answer that can help settle the inner tension, often by enabling you to put things in perspective and to integrate the other needs and voices.

The Meaning Maker is not a distant, remote source of wisdom, like some inner Yoda who must be sought after in distant realms for his answers. This part of your personality is involved in almost every decision, and its wisdom is particularly valuable when all the other subpersonalities have weighed in.

On the other hand, just as Yoda urges the young Luke Skywalker to be patient in his quest to learn the ways of the Jedi Knights in *Star Wars,* the Meaning Maker favors a long deliberative process, rather than instant gratification and easy answers. If you make snap, impetuous decisions all the time, you may not be giving this part of your personality the opportunity to offer you the benefit of its counsel.

If you find yourself asking questions like the ones that follow, chances are your Meaning Maker is hard at work. Note that specific questions such as these often lead to more questions, ones that are strategic and even bigger picture in nature (shown in italics in the following examples). This tendency to "zoom out" is a characteristic of the Meaning Maker. "This is the part of us that deepens and broadens the question and asks us to consider a wider horizon of possibilities and consequences," says Coach Meg.

WHEN YOU ASK: "Is this marriage going to work out?"
NEXT ASK YOURSELF: *"What is the larger lesson or meaning of my marital challenges? How is this experience asking me to grow?"*

WHEN YOU ASK: "Is taking this job the right decision?"
NEXT ASK YOURSELF: *"How will this job decision impact my life five years from now? What new adventures might the job bring that will open up new horizons down the road?"*

WHEN YOU ASK: "Should I try to adopt a vegan diet?"
NEXT ASK YOURSELF: *"How will I know whether a vegan diet is healthier for my body? What signs might I watch out for?"*

When you ask: "Should I accept the transfer to the West Coast office?"

Next ask yourself: "*How would a transfer to the West Coast office impact my well-being, my family's well-being? What contribution to my career would the move make? Which matters most at this stage of my life?*"

When you ask: "Do I switch majors?"

Next ask yourself: "*What major inspires and interests me the most in the short term? What major would be more likely to lead to the best career opportunities in the long term? What is the best decision right now?*"

When you ask: "Do I go back to school to try something completely new?"

Next ask yourself: "*Would I make better use of my talents if I were to go back to school and gain the basis and the confidence for a new career track? Would that satisfy more of my needs than what I'm doing now?*"

When you ask: "Should I take piano lessons?"

Next ask yourself: "*What are the pros and cons of learning to play the piano? What kind of investment would I have to make in piano lessons, how much time would they entail, and would the eventual pleasure I derive from musical expression and this adventure in learning about the piano and piano theory and music outweigh these initial expenditures? Can I commit to the practice time needed to achieve proficiency, and if so, how would I have to reorder my schedule or reprioritize my activities?*"

The future is uncertain. Life, and the decisions we make as we move through it, is often not black and white, but is fraught with ambiguity. Indeed, we spend a lot of our lives living with the questions, *not* getting answers. The Meaning Maker helps us see that that is okay, that there is growth even out of not knowing, and that recognizing whether a course of action is the right or wrong one may be evident only in the fullness of time, if ever.

"Good coaches help people tune in to and listen to their Meaning Maker for inner guidance and wisdom," says Coach Meg. "It's basically an inner coach!"

1. What role does the Meaning Maker play in my life, and how has it shaped me?

Everyone experiences the Meaning Maker differently. For some, it's the cooler head. For others, it's the arbitrator, building compromise among the battling factions of your Inner Family. In its acceptance and tolerance of other points of view, it may be the source of what Lincoln called "the better angels of our nature."

The Meaning Maker might have been there at a time when you needed to make a big decision. Perhaps after much handwringing and inner turmoil, you finally came to a conclusion and said to yourself, *Okay, this is what I'm going to do. . . .* Well, that decisive moment probably followed the weighing in of your Meaning Maker.

Let's say you've lost your job. You're in crisis mode. The Meaning Maker is the subpersonality that can help you see how this job loss might be a good thing, an opportunity to reinvent yourself, a way to break out of a rut or an unhappy situation. It's also the subpersonality that helps you put it all in perspective, so that you can see the bigger picture, the silver lining.

The Meaning Maker was probably involved when you made a decision about college, about your partner, about where to live, and about what to do with your life. But it's also there guiding you day to day, if you invite its insights.

"It's not just for the big decisions," says Coach Meg. "You're about to yell at your child, but the Meaning Maker puts a hand on your shoulder and says, 'Is a screaming match going to solve anything?' It helps you tame the frenzy."

Where there is chaos in your life, the Meaning Maker can bring a little order and light.

In fact, Meg considers it her Inner Coach. "Every single morning the Meaning Maker gives me words of wisdom for the day ahead," she says.

It can do the same for you, too. If you're listening.

2. What story best captures the Meaning Maker's biggest contribution to my life?

Here's one that may resonate with many. Coach Meg worked with an ambitious entrepreneur who prided himself on his initiative and responsiveness. He was adept at making decisions quickly and pushing forward to forge new business ground. The downside was a constant frustration and impatience, because of his sense that the rest of the world moved more slowly, and thus his business didn't grow as quickly as it ought to given his prodigious efforts. Once Meg taught him to consult his Meaning Maker quietly each morning, the entrepreneur gained the ability to let things go, to proceed at his own pace. As his Meaning Maker counseled, among other things, patience and acceptance, he could then replace the frenzy of frustration with equanimity, freeing

up emotional energy for creative tasks. A simple serenity p
("Change what you can, accept what you can't change, and ac
the wisdom to know the difference") became a daily touchstor
and he continues to use it in his successful career.

3. On a scale of 1–10, how well are the Meaning Maker's needs being met today, and how important are those needs to my well-being?

A lot of people aren't regularly tuning in to their Meaning Maker. Coach Meg believes that one reason why the inner dialogue can be so messy and why so many people feel as if their lives are in such turmoil is that they haven't availed themselves of this capacity. Why not? Well, it's hard to reach. It takes a little time and patience. It's not a noisy voice; it doesn't often make quick, assertive decisions.

The Meaning Maker is best consulted in quiet places, where there is no distraction, and when you can take time to stop and listen. Ever wonder why so many people come back from a vacation and announce that they're going to make a change in this or that aspect of their life? Part of it stems from the chance to relax, sure. But part of it is that when we have time off from our day-to-day routines (and stressors), we have the time to tune in to the Meaning Maker.

Now if you'd like to book a trip to the Caribbean as an excuse to listen to your Meaning Maker, bon voyage! But you don't have to go on vacation—in fact, you don't really have to go anywhere—to put yourself in a position to listen to it. Runners, walkers, hikers, cyclists—people who are out on their own, often

, engaged in rhythmic exercise activities where
ɹr bodies on cruise control and let their thoughts
ɹ themselves accessing their Meaning Maker, while
ɹhening their cardiovascular system. Similarly, those
ɹtice meditation or sit quietly in a church pew or just rest
ɹr living-room couch can access it, too.

4. What can I do to better meet the needs of the Meaning Maker?

You have to hit the PAUSE button in your life. For just a few seconds, gently pull your mind back from the inner and outer noise, nudge the dial down on the constant chatter and distractions, and dial in to this voice. As just noted, you can do that when you're lying on a beach, walking down a trail, kneeling in a pew, or simply sitting in your living room, breathing deeply.

Whenever you find the time to tune out the internal and external distractions, you're able to tune in to the Meaning Maker, which often gives you the calm, clear-thinking, wise perspective you need. The Meaning Maker is oftentimes the source of solutions. Of course, because it is a part of you, these are *your* solutions—not insights delivered from some other realm. They are the result of a synthesis of the other perspectives voiced in our often frenetic inner dialogues. The calm, logical perspective that this capacity in humans seems capable of delivering is often the last word on a problem. So why, you may ask, do so many people remain mired in their problems or make bad and illogical decisions? They simply might not take the time to hit that PAUSE button. They might not even know where it is on their inner remote.

THE MEANING MAKER, CASE BY CASE

In previous chapters, we used case studies from Coach Meg's practice to illustrate the inner dialogue and the conflicts that can arise between different voices. Each of the case studies included a Roll Call, in which every one of the nine subpersonalities was allowed to voice its side of the issue that these individuals were grappling with. Did you notice that the Meaning Maker was always the last one we asked in our Roll Calls? There's a reason for that. The other subpersonalities can't settle down until they are heard, so they clamor for your attention. Once all the members of your Inner Family, all the emotions and needs, have been welcomed and have expressed themselves, then and only then can you turn to the wise counsel, the Meaning Maker.

We concluded each of the case studies by telling you how the individuals ended up resolving their struggles. The solutions weren't always ideal or perfect; very often they were compromises. "But they were sensible and actionable, and in most of the cases," Coach Meg says, "these individuals were satisfied with the solutions." And although she might have helped nudge things along in the right direction, the solutions, the answers to these people's problems, ultimately came from within once the wise counsel of the Meaning Maker had been accessed.

Let's go back and review these case studies so you can see the critical role this subpersonality played in some of them—and how it can help you in your decision making.

The conflict for **Laura**, twenty-four, our case study for Autonomy, was that she wanted to make a radical change in her life and move to South America. Autonomy and her Curious Adventurer were pushing for this. The others weren't so sure. The Meaning

Maker essentially advised the Curious Adventurer, "Hey, this is great energy, and it's a positive instinct to want to seek these new horizons. However, this may not be the ideal time in life to make such a drastic move. Let's come up with other adventures that would satisfy the need for new experiences."

Facilitating this communication among subpersonalities, which Laura articulated during her session with Coach Meg, is an important function of the Meaning Maker. "It has the ability to listen without judgment to the other parts," says Coach Meg. "Remember that these voices can be seen as the inner expressions of all our emotions, signaling all our needs. The Meaning Maker is a higher-level capacity that really respects and listens before offering wisdom."

Bobby, the firefighter, wasn't listening to his Body Regulator. He was eating poorly and was sedentary. Moreover, as he had just been promoted to lieutenant, his Relational capacity had shifted: he had gone from being one of the guys to being the guy in charge. His Meaning Maker helped mediate between these two voices, essentially helping Bobby's Relational see that it needed to mature and grow up, and that part of that process entailed leading by example in terms of healthy behaviors.

Jason, twenty-one, and his mother, **Elizabeth,** fifty-two, came to Coach Meg together. Elizabeth, a successful attorney, wanted Jason to follow in her and her husband's footsteps and apply to law school. But Jason's Roll Call was unanimous in the desire to strike a different path. He was passionate about and committed to becoming a teacher, as he felt he could help mold young minds. "I'm a different person, and I have different goals," his Autonomy asserted. Given that he was a young man, Jason's unanimity of purpose—and voices—suggested a Meaning Maker wise beyond its years. Whatever inner conflicts Jason had had about not following in his parents' career footsteps had long since been resolved by the time he and his mother visited Coach Meg.

And when Elizabeth heard what her son had to reveal, she realized she was wrong to try to deter him. "By the time I heard Jason's Meaning Maker, I realized how much this idea of becoming a teacher really matters to him," she said.

For **Mary,** sixty-one, who lived a perhaps too-comfortable, predictable life, the inner lines were more sharply drawn: her Autonomy, Creative, and Curious Adventurer all wanted change. The other subpersonalities were against it. In this case, the Meaning Maker, pointing out she was now at the age when time became a more precious commodity, advocated for the three proponents of change—all of them voices that had been ignored in the past. "The Meaning Maker helped to bring those parts alive," Coach Meg says. But again, the Meaning Maker didn't prompt Mary to do anything rash and radical. She decided to make some small but meaningful changes, without completely upending her ordered life, which helped satisfy all.

Jeanine and **Kevin,** an engaged couple in their early thirties, seemed like polar opposites. She was structured, organized, risk averse. He was a dreamer. And he was bad with deadlines and appointments, and was impossible when it came to keeping a neat office, but he was very creative and was always looking for something new—like that risky new career as a writer of crime fiction he wanted to embark on. On the surface, it appeared that they were people driven by very different things and that each lacked attributes the other seemed endowed with.

The standard advice might have been, "You just have to accept your differences." But in this case, both Jeanine's and Kevin's Meaning Makers, after listening and reflecting, realized something else. Here's exactly what their Meaning Makers said at the conclusion of their joint Roll Call:

> *Jeanine:* "Being with him is going to provide a voice for my Creative, which is being stifled. I know I need that, despite the Executive Manager's reservations, and that's a good balance for me."
>
> *Kevin:* "If I want to meet my goal, if I want to make a go of it as an author, on my own, I admit I need to get a little bit more structure. I have the capability to do it. I just have to listen to it more."

Both of them did make efforts to work on their "weaknesses"—or, in the parlance of the Inner Family, to give their less dominant capacities more opportunity to express themselves. So Jeanine allowed her Creative to engage in some more spontaneous behavior; Kevin gave his Executive Manager more attention and the authority to structure his life a little more.

There were no cases more challenging than that of seventy-six-year-old **Florence,** who had to negotiate her needs not only with her various subpersonalities but also with her forty-one-year-old son, **Martin,** who encouraged her to consult Coach Meg. "Florence had a lot of conflicts," says Coach Meg. "She wanted more independence, but she also wanted to be more connected with her son, who felt she needed to be living in a more structured environment . . . and essentially had to give up some of that independence for what he perceived was her own good."

During Florence's Roll Call, it became apparent that each part of her wanted something different. Autonomy didn't want to move into a senior residence; the Curious Adventurer wanted more energy and activity; the Body Regulator wanted more exercise and social contact; the Relational lamented the loss of old friends. "You had a lot of agendas," Coach Meg says. "The Meaning Maker played the role of synthesizer here, and it managed to address many perspectives together in a complex stage of life."

Florence's Meaning Maker came up with a new mind-set, resolving first that, while she loved her son and appreciated his concern, it would be for her to decide when the time had come to sell her house and move into a senior-living facility; and second, that she would forge a new way of life, making a conscious effort to reengage socially with some old friends and to find some new ones. This included visiting a friend in a senior community, where Florence planned to join her for a weekly exercise class geared to older adults.

It was a solution for which the Meaning Maker addressed and delicately balanced the needs of all the subpersonalities and one son. Says Coach Meg, "It shows the capability of this capability!"

CASE STUDY:
The Meaning Maker

DR. EDDIE: Dr. Dan, age fifty-three

Dr. Dan Witkowski pulled me aside at a medical conference for a quick "curbside" consultation. (That's doctors' lingo for informal help on a clinical question.) He was an ob-gyn, so I was wondering how my training in physical medicine and rehabilitation would be of value to his work, but of course, I was happy to assist a colleague, particularly one as exuberant and likeable as Dan.

"Who's the patient?" I inquired.

"Me. My muscles are really sore now that I have started weight lifting. Maybe I should already know, but please reassure me. Is that normal?"

"Yes. You'll get used to it as you continue to exercise. It's called delayed onset muscle soreness, DOMS for short, and it's fine as long as your joints don't hurt. By the way, what got you to start lifting weights?"

"I'm hoping that getting stronger will help me keep up on the soccer field," he explained.

I inquired just a bit more deeply. "You're right. Weight lifting will probably help, but what got you back into soccer?"

I am always working with my patients to motivate them to become more active and take on resistance training as part of their self-care, so when I run into someone who is starting or is already physically active, I like to ask what got them going. I always learn something that may help someone else (or sometimes even me!). It usually takes a bit of digging to find the true motivation for change.

Dan paused for a moment, broke eye contact, drew a deep breath, and regained his composure. "It's because of my dad," he said, quickly adding, "But I'm doing it for my own family and for myself." He pulled out of his pocket a well-worn leather wallet and produced a picture of himself and his overweight, but beaming dad, a clearly proud father standing by his accomplished son. In the picture, his dad was holding an oversize lobster, which he appeared to be about to devour with great relish. I started thinking about my choices for dinner tonight, but Dan brought me back to attention.

"This is his wallet," he said. "I've carried it every day since he died from a massive heart attack three years ago. He was only seventy-five. It was all preventable." From the wallet, he pulled out a small square of paper and unfolded it. On the creased sheet of paper were eighteen neatly typed medications to treat his dad's high blood pressure, high cholesterol, and high blood sugar, and to treat the side effects of those very medications.

"He was such a good patient," Dan said sadly, looking at the list. "He took every pill his doctors prescribed for him. But no one ever helped him to start exercising, change his diet, or lose weight to avoid the heart attack that killed him." He looked back at me. "Think about it, Eddie. When we were in medical school, we were never taught anything about nutrition or the value of exercise. I mean, it wasn't a field of study!"

He's right, I thought. And I'm a good example of that. I remember only one lecture on nutrition.

"After Dad died, I realized it was time for me to take some action," Dan continued. "So I started reading up on diet and fitness, and I've decided to become a vegetarian to improve my health, and I've started exercising. Then I read about the importance of strength training to maintain quality of life when you get older . . . and, well, here I am."

My simple question had led to Dan easily revealing a powerful Meaning Maker in his life. His dad's death, a clear reminder of his own mortality, and his strong desire not to leave his own six children without a dad were compelling reasons for Dan to make multiple significant changes in his life.

"Has it been difficult changing your diet and starting the exercise routine?" I asked and then witnessed Dan's recounting of his own Inner Family dynamics. His actual family was highest on the list for Dan, so he started there.

"Some of our family members don't quite get it, and I don't want to offend them, so at Easter I do have our family's traditional meal of kielbasa and pierogi," he said. "It's almost sacrilegious not to in the Witkowski house, and truth be told, I really still love those foods. But my kids and my wife are supportive. Pam has become a vegetarian, as well. That's really helped me stick with it, and I'm so proud of her."

Clearly, Dan's strong Relational voice had listened to the counsel of the powerful Meaning Maker.

I continued my inquiry. "What's has been the toughest part of changing your lifestyle?"

"I'm pretty good at structuring my time and running my practice. I grew up playing soccer, so joining a team and getting back on the field was a no-brainer. The weight lifting is a bit more of a challenge, but I like how quickly I am getting stronger. I like to cook, so I look at learning some meat-free recipes as a creative exercise." He paused, and I could almost see a thought balloon with a honey ham, fresh out of the oven, hovering over his head. "Eddie, I'll be honest. It's hard changing the habits you've developed over a lifetime. But whenever I'm thinking I want to blow off the gym, or I get the urge for a double cheeseburger with a side of fries, I just fish out my dad's wallet. It keeps me on target."

I could sense that Dan's Executive Manager was reorganizing his schedule and that his Creative voice was participating in the new menu. I also thought his Curious Adventurer might be pushing him toward trying other forms of physical activity, as well as new ways of eating. That was all healthy, in every sense of the word.

Before I finished hearing from Dan's entire Inner Family, he diverted attention from himself.

"So, Eddie, what drives you? I see you biking to work. You seem pretty good at taking care of yourself. What's your secret?"

With the tables turned, I thought about the role my own

Meaning Maker played in this and how the rest of my Inner Family had got with the program.

"The simple answer is that I've made it a habit. I work out regularly, and I try to eat well, and I feel better as a result. But"—and here I confided to Dan, and now I'm confiding to you, some more profound truths than I would if I struck up a conversation with the person on the elliptical machine next to me at the gym—"on a deeper level, I'm thinking about my kids, too. And about my patients. I'm thinking, Dan, I'd like to be a good role model for them in every way . . . but particularly in the way I take care of myself as I get older. I want them to see that not everybody who's over forty has to be overweight and out of shape and taking a lot of medication. I want to show people that even with a busy schedule, it's possible. And I like to practice what I preach."

"Wow," said Dan as I realized this was becoming quite the curbside consult. "That's great. Well, thanks for the advice."

"Keep up the good work," I told him before we went our separate ways. "Remember, change is hard, but it is easier with a big goal in mind."

He just smiled and nodded as he patted the wallet in his pocket. Dan's Meaning Maker had provided a powerful reason for him to change his lifestyle, and the rest of his Inner Family had gotten with the program.

How do you find the Meaning Maker in your life? By digging a bit to find the "why behind the why." This will make any change more sustainable, as it will be attached to a bigger purpose. Dan's first answer to the question of why he had started lifting weights was that he wanted to become more competitive on the soccer field. It took just a bit more digging to uncover a much more powerful motivation: Dan's connection to his dad and his children. Being aware of the true, deeper motivation for an action or a change will help keep you on course better than the more superficial reason for it.

The Meaning Maker can help articulate the clear purpose for any action or change, and this will align the rest of your Inner Family and draw other people to support your purpose and the work of adopting and sustaining meaningful change in your life.

11

THE MAXIMS OF MULTIPLICITY

In this book, you've learned about the concept of the Inner Family, essentially the idea that our psyche has discrete entities, otherwise known as aspects, parts, or subpersonalities, among other terms, that come together, ideally in harmony, in the way we interact with the world.

When someone says, usually in reference to the members of a group of people, that "they are of one mind on this issue," it means that after some debate and discussion, presumably, the group members have reached a consensus. A similar process happens in the mind of each of us as individuals. Every one of us experiences this multiplicity of mind, that is, multiple points of view that exist separately, whether we consciously recognize it or not. In our day-to-day life none of us (the exception being, of course, those who have been exposed to the ideas presented in this book) walk around saying, "Hey, you know what my Executive Manager is telling me? I shouldn't be going out to the movies to-night, when I have so much work to do!" We do not remark, "My

Autonomy is saying, 'When's the last time you did something you really wanted to do?'"

We don't conceive of ourselves as having a mind with such parts. We don't walk around thinking that we necessarily have these different voices in our head. Consequently, we often fail to recognize that what we hear in that incessant internal monologue often comes from different and sometimes competing places and needs.

Through the Roll Calls and the case studies in this book, we've shown that there's great value in pausing to tune in to each of those different parts of ourselves, essentially zeroing in and consulting each separately, and then letting them come back together more harmoniously to help us make better decisions or reduce the stress and the frenzy in our lives and thrive.

Now that you realize you have these different subpersonalities, and now that you've learned how you can tease them out and listen to them one at a time, let's look at how this theory of multiplicity can be put into practice in your day-to-day life.

Doing so means accepting a few truths, some of them a bit harsh.

First, it's complicated. *You're* complicated. All human beings are. It's valuable to accept this and to recognize that there are going to be things in life that come up for which we are not prepared. The unpredictable circumstances in life can trigger reactions from this complicated network within us, and that can immediately throw out of whack the balance we may have achieved just a moment ago.

That said—and this is our second truth—while these inherent competing drives are part of being human, so is the ability to achieve a balance and compromise. Just as groups, organizations, and countries can hammer out agreements and treaties, so, too, can you establish order and equanimity among the different aspects of your personality. Not in perpetuity. Not for all time. But at least enough of the time to make your life calmer and more fulfilling.

How do you do this? How do you know that you are making the right choices when you are being pushed and pulled in different directions by the inner dynamics of your competing needs? How do you integrate your subpersonalities in a way that brings you to a state of equanimity and calm? One way is by recognizing and accepting five principles, or as we call them, the Maxims of Multiplicity.

THE MAXIMS OF MULTIPLICITY: PRINCIPLES TO KEEP IN MIND FOR MASTERING YOUR MULTIPLICITY OF MIND

If you are going to shift to viewing yourself as having multiplicity of mind, you should have a solid understanding of the principles of living your life with this new self-awareness.

Recognize that it's always something

There are always going to be inner conflicts. You've heard the term *creative tension*? It's usually used to describe the healthy push and pull between talented people, artists, or innovators who work collectively to create something. But it applies here, as well. Your instinct for order (the Executive Manager) and routine (the Body Regulator) are always going to be pushing and pulling to some degree against your need for excitement and change (the Curious Adventurer). We've seen this tension, with varying degrees of intensity, in the different scenarios in all the case studies in this book, and you are now probably aware of it within yourself. Acceptance of all of what makes you, well, *you* is a key step toward you being able to navigate your internal dialogue with more ease.

Check the forecast!

We have taught you that there are at least nine discrete aspects of your personality, based upon core needs common to all. We've also shown how, when they are in harmony and balance, you thrive. When they are in conflict, life can be messy and difficult. And, as we showed through our case studies, when you listen to each of them, you can often find a way to reach a compromise, pull them together as an Inner Family, and move forward. Sometimes that compromise can be as fragile as a temporary cease-fire between constantly warring nations. While you may be able to reach a consensus or at least a balance when dealing with a life issue or an imminent decision, remember that really understanding your inner self (or selves) requires a regular process of consultation.

You have an emotional weather report that changes as fast as the weather. This isn't about being "moody." It's about an ongoing reappraisal and reevaluation of how your different needs are being met in the ongoing rush of life's events. The emotional weather report is rarely as definitive as, say, the high and low temperature predictions in a meteorological forecast. For most of us, few days are 100 percent sunny, and few days bring torrential rain that falls from dawn until dusk. It's usually partly cloudy or partly sunny in the forecast of your mind, with a couple parts feeling good, one part feeling soggy, and one part downcast. And you can have all that happening at once.

But through the Roll Call, which we showed you how to do

earlier, you can take apart your emotional weather report and use that at any point to decode your emotional state, a mix of feelings, and better understand why you feel the way you do at any given moment, and how you might improve your internal weather. It takes only a few moments.

Appreciate the contributions

We must go beyond being simply aware of our subpersonalities. This is the step when we acknowledge that each of the different parts of our personalities makes a valuable contribution to the whole, just as many orchestra sections contribute to a symphony. This is about listening and acknowledging that your Curious Adventurer feels stifled, and that's important, because it is this part of you that is the primary motivator for getting you to try new things. Or maybe it's that your Relational is sad. It's usually good at reaching out to people you care about for support, but perhaps it is temporarily unable to. That may explain why you've been feeling alone with your blues. It could be that your Meaning Maker is raising questions that you're not giving it the space to try to answer, and maybe that's why you have this vague sense that professionally, you're stagnant and going nowhere. All these parts, these subpersonalities, are important; all of them play key roles in helping you thrive, but first you have to acknowledge them and appreciate them and allow them fuller expression.

Keep it in perspective

We just discussed the value of each subpersonality and how each should be appreciated for its contributions. The inverse of that is not letting one subpersonality run the show or ruin your entire outlook.

When you say to yourself, *I'm upset,* and you realize it's actually just one part of yourself that's upset, the feeling seems a little more manageable. It helps to understand that it's not all of you that's in distress, just a part of you. That way, it doesn't seem so overwhelming. Remember that within you there are nine perspectives on almost every issue. Don't let one drag all the rest down!

Get yourself together!

Just as we shouldn't let one voice, one need out of nine dominate our life in a negative way, so, too, should we recognize that galvanizing our Inner Family, pulling all these subpersonalities together as a unified team, free of nagging doubts and dissent, can be an enormously powerful asset. As we've seen, sometimes one aspect of our personality can be too shrill, too dominant when asserting its needs. The underlying need being expressed is not "wrong," and therefore, if you can find a way to heed what that voice is saying and harmonize it with the rest of the voices (as was done in the Roll Calls in our case studies), you can find yourself in a very formidable position in life, able to tackle whatever comes your way. That's when you're acting with single-minded purposiveness.

In the next section are some ideas on how and when to use these powerful discoveries you've made about yourself in daily life.

USING THE MULTIPLICITY OF MIND IN DAY-TO-DAY LIFE

If you've ever embarked on an exercise program, you know that one of the things you're encouraged to do, in order to make sure you're not trying to progress too far, too fast, is to "listen to your body." Pulling together and harnessing the power of your Inner Family requires something similar, except we're asking you to listen to the different aspects of yourself. You probably have no trouble recognizing that a sore leg, a winded state, sweating, and panting are all distinct physiological signs from various parts of your body that you're pushing yourself hard, maybe a little too hard. Deciphering the inner expressions of your needs is a little trickier.

However, at this point, as you've learned about your multiplicity of mind, you may have some sense of which of your voices have been dominant, which have been stifled, and how that has affected your decision making and your life's path up to this point.

Another way to look at this is to recognize that you've got capabilities that haven't been fully tapped. So now that you know they're in there, let's use them to help you manage better in life and thrive.

To help you move from internal chaos to equanimity

Equanimity entails a state of balance, composure, coolness, and evenness of temper. It's the exact opposite of the stressed-out frenzy that most twenty-first-century people seem to find themselves in. Blame it on the speed of digital technology and technological change, blame it on the complexities of modern life, or blame it on too many stimuli or too much caffeine. Whatever the cause of this frenzy, one antidote to it is touching base with yourself: you can move to that state of equanimity and composure—even for just brief periods of time—by checking in with your Inner Family.

For this exercise, you can use the four questions posed in preceding chapters to tune in to each member of your Inner Family and decode your emotions (What role does this subpersonality play in my life, and how has it shaped me? What story best captures its biggest contribution to my life? On a scale of 1–10, how well are its needs being met today, and how important are those needs to my well-being? What can I do to better meet the needs of this subpersonality?)

Or you can approach your Inner Family as a whole—like at a board meeting—and pose a single question to all the members. For example, that question might be "What are we doing about this move to California I've been contemplating?" Allow each part of yourself to weigh in. You will probably hear some passionate arguments for why you should move to California and some practical reasons for why you shouldn't—and vice versa.

If your Creative and your Curious Adventurer are dominant voices, they may argue loudly for such a move. But if you don't heed the others' perspectives, you may find yourself waking up one morning in Los Angeles and saying, "I'm unhappy. Why did I do this?" And that might be because voices that weren't heeded during the decision-making process are now expressing their displeasure. And now you're hearing your Relational say, "We've got no friends in California. I'm lonely," and your Body Regulator lament, "Life is a roller coaster here. Nothing is settled, and stress is sky high." If you'd allowed room for these perspectives in the debate before you made the move, you might have still moved, but you would have strategized and planned to meet some of the needs of the subpersonalities that weren't happy with the move.

In other words, if you had calmly "roundtabled" the question in your mind, you would have arrived at a more thorough internal picture and a better sense of the pros and cons of the move and what it could (or might not) do for you, from the point of view of all your emotions and needs. Whatever decision you arrived at would have been one in which you were truly vested—every part of you!

By incorporating each of your inner perspectives in the decision-making process, you don't guarantee that you will make the right decision, but you do assure yourself a measure of peace of mind, of equanimity.

To help you resolve a work or personal crisis

Let's say somebody has angered you at work by taking credit for something that you did, credit that you were deserving of. The boss seems to have accepted the coworker's claims that she did the good work. Now she is getting the praise, while you get zip.

It's not an earth-shaking thing that will negatively affect your career, but it still stings. So you take a deep breath, step back from the situation, and as calmly as possible try to tune in (or tease out) the reactions of your different inner voices. Here's what your emotional weather forecast map shows you:

Autonomy feels like crap. ("This was something I'd been charged with. I was doing a great job, and now they've taken it away from me.")

Confidence is soggier than a summer afternoon in Florida. ("I'm sad because obviously no one thinks I'm capable of doing this. Everyone assumed that the other person was right in taking the credit, because they couldn't imagine that I would be able to do the work she claimed to have done.")

And Relational feels betrayed. ("I thought I could trust this person.")

You figure out that it's really these three subpersonalities that got stepped on. They're the ones feeling most hurt. Other subpersonalities offer their unique perspective. Your Meaning Maker points out that you've known for months that this coworker was insecure about her job and about herself. She did this as a way to make herself feel better, to justify her own position in the company.

That's a good point. You mull that over. Now you've gone from feeling slighted and angry to having a clearer understanding of what you're feeling (and also of what the offending party feels). You feel better after realizing all that! Now, from a calmer perspective, you can figure out a course of action.

You decide, with the help of the Meaning Maker, that perhaps this is not, as the saying goes, your hill to die on. You decide it's really not worth a fight. The Standard Setter says, "Keep doing good work. It will eventually be recognized." And the Relational might say, "Hey, I should pay attention to what other people are doing . . . and give credit where credit is due. It's important to be grateful to other people. We know how it feels when they're not grateful to us!"

What you've done in this instance is move from internal chaos to equanimity simply by acknowledging and listening to and decoding each of your emotions. Try it next time you're angry over something. See if just stepping back and listening to the different perspectives expressed within you doesn't help clarify and defuse the situation—while also providing a solution.

To help you address other life questions, big or small

You're deciding whether to take a new job or enter into a relationship, whether to join the PTA or a gardening club, or whether or not to work on improving your golf game.

You can consult your subpersonalities and find out if any of these options is going to work. Let's take, in this case, the less dramatic example of improving your golf game. The Standard Setter wants you to work on your game so that you're able to play as well as your buddies. Improving your game also wouldn't hurt professionally: it would mean that the next time the boss or one of your clients invites you to a charity match or for an afternoon on the links, you wouldn't have to come up with some lame excuse for why you couldn't be there.

But the Relational then says, "If you go golfing this weekend, you'll be gone all day, and you won't see the kids. Your wife won't be happy, and the kids barely get to see you as it is, given your work schedule lately."

Knowing this, you prioritize and realize that you have to be a father first, one of the guys second. But you decide that what you'll do with your kids is take them to the driving range (okay, if they're really young, maybe it's miniature golf). That way you're addressing the Relational. But maybe while you're at the range with the kids, you'll get to practice your swing, which will please the Standard Setter, so that next time you do play golf with the guys, you won't look like a complete amateur. If you ignore the Relational or the Standard Setter—or if you are oblivious to the whole idea that you have these parts of you expressing your needs—you might make a decision based on the most pressing need at the moment.

That's often what happens, as we've seen in the case studies. We make decisions based on the loudest voices in our inner dialogue. What we need to do is take a Roll Call and convene the entire Inner Family and really begin to hear what the other voices have to say.

To help you better understand and relate to others

The Inner Family approach is not only a way to better understand yourself; it can also help you gain insight into the behavior of others. By recognizing that your spouse, your children, your parents, your boss, coworkers, and friends are all listening to their own chorus of voices and needs, you gain valuable insight into others' behavior, intentions, and emotional reactions. That is a valuable tool for better communications and better relationships.

How do you recognize and work with others' Inner Families? We would like to close our book with Dr. Eddie's last case study, which revolves around his own family's interactions. We think it's an inspiring example of how the Inner Family concept can be applied in real life, and help you and your loved ones thrive.

DR. EDDIE:
We Are Famil(ies)

As I gathered with my family at the kitchen table, I heard my family members projecting their own dominant voices into the dinner conversation.

My son, the entrepreneurial, hilarious, out-of-the-box thinker, was imagining and describing the future of the Internet and how his nascent app company could capitalize on this. His Creative voice was undeterred by practical considerations, and his Executive Manager seemed late to the party (as he had been to dinner).

Our middle daughter was describing her plans for her gap year before college and was chagrined that registration had not yet opened for a volunteer program in Europe nine months from now. She was ready to sign up today. Her Executive Manager organized her time, her thinking, and often the family's activities. She interrupted her brother's flurry of creative ideas and directed us back to discussing the plans for our family vacation. Years earlier, she had looked at her brother and had asked me to help her become funnier, like he was. Indeed, using her dominant Executive Manager, she had set out a plan to work at her own humor and had since developed her own timing and wit.

Meanwhile, our youngest daughter sat at the table, doodling on her wrist with a pen. She struggled to overcome the dominant voices of her older siblings at the table, her quieter voice waiting to get a word in. She listened intently and then spoke up to offer her more blended voices, reflecting on a book about a dystopian society, which she'd read last night, instead of doing her biology project.

As my wife and I raise our children—Jesse, twenty; Becca, eighteen; and Aliza, fifteen—I am reminded that as with our individual inner voices, the dinner table Roll Call needs to go beyond labeling and pigeonholing one child as creative and the next as organized. Indeed, I was at first incredulous that our disorganized, creative son was put in charge of logistics for part of a group trip to Central America and then was elected as a freshman to become social chair of his college fraternity.

So as we passed the chicken and vegetables one night, I decided to ask him and his siblings about it, to prompt a somewhat unsolicited Roll Call of my own kids, starting with Mr. Creative.

"How is it that you routinely lose your wallet and are often late or miss appointments altogether, but you were able to coordinate and direct a daylong festival for hundreds of college students?" I asked him.

"It's all about the group, Dad," he replied. "I guess it's just not that important to me as an individual to always be on time, but no one else in the fraternity was stepping up, so I felt I had to. I guess I can get organized if it is important enough to me."

Listening to my son, I could hear his Relational voice rallying the rest of his voices and literally waking up the Executive Manager. "We've got a show to put on! We can't let my 'brothers' down. Yes, I know you detest making lists, but find a pen and paper and stop complaining."

Amazed by our middle daughter's ability to manage complex tasks, I was reminded similarly not to discount Becca's quieter but present Creative voice.

"You are so methodical and organized in your schoolwork, exercise, and violin practice. Do you think this squashes your creativity?"

"Dad, you've been hearing me practice classical violin pieces for years," she reminded me. "Sure, that takes discipline, but my real creative side comes out when I play fiddle music by ear and wing it in a group. It's kind of like when I get everything organized to follow a recipe from a cookbook and then let my imagination lead me to change the recipe just to see how it will taste. So I guess being organized allows me to be more creative."

Meanwhile our youngest sat at the table, now rearranging her vegetables into an abstract cityscape. Her Creative reigned, while her Executive Manager spoke in a quiet voice and needed a good kick in the pants to get active. She had been characteristically silent as she listened to her two older siblings explain their Inner Families. I turned to her.

"I know you put off that math assignment until the last minute. But you got it done, and you got an A minus," I said as she made a face. "How did you organize yourself to get it done in time?"

"Well," Aliza said, shooting me a look to remind me that she'd still rather be doodling than having to explain things to me, "I'd much rather be trying out my new colored pencils. But I know I have to get good grades. So I kind of set a goal for myself, and then it's a bit easier to get myself organized."

Her Standard Setter had been just the encouragement that her Executive Manager needed for her to wake (with three alarms).

Needless to say, it was an instructive dinner, and my wife, Alison, and I came away not only feeling prouder of our three kids, but also having the odd feeling that there were five people but at least ten voices at the dinner table . . . all with something important to say.

Dr. Eddie and Alison have learned to appreciate the Inner Family within each of the members of their actual family. We hope that what we have presented in this book will help you do the same with yours, as well. We realize we may have stretched the limits of your imagination with the very concept of the Inner Family and the multiplicity of mind. But when you can truly discern these parts of your psyche, give them the opportunity to have voices, they absolutely come alive and impart a great deal of wisdom. Of course, it's all you in the end, but we hope that through appreciating your multiplicity of mind, *you* will find a multiplicity of new ways to lead a more fulfilling, productive, happy life and to thrive.

ACKNOWLEDGMENTS

We would like to thank the former and current editors in chief at Harvard Health Publications (HHP)—Julie Silver, MD, and Gregory Curfman, MD, respectively—for their support of this book. Also, our literary agent, Linda Konner, and our editor, Deb Brody, both of whom guided us wisely through our second HHP book, and first for William Morrow.

The great thinkers whose ideas form the basis of the book are cited in our sources, and we'd like to offer special thanks to Carol Kauffman, Dick Schwartz, and Katherine Peil for their contributions and inspiration.

Margaret is grateful to her husband, Paul Clark, a biotechnology patent attorney, for codeveloping an evolutionary narrative for the nine human capacities.

Margaret and Eddie wish to thank their colleagues, coaches, and patients, each of whom in their own way has helped them enjoy and appreciate the diversity, inherent conflicts, and occasionally beautiful harmony of being human.

John would like to thank his colleagues at the New York Institute of Technology for their ongoing support of his writing, particularly Vice President of Academic Affairs Rahmat Shoureshi and Dean James Simon.

Special thanks from us all to Dan Witkowski, MD, and to the Phillips family for allowing their stories to be shared; to the folks at NASA, in particular Jeremy Eggers and Bill Wroebel, for granting us permission to use Clara Ma's wonderful essay on curiosity; to Kristin Lindstrom for her assistance on research; and to the late Dean Kujala for helping us to visualize the Inner Family and our multiplicity of mind.

Finally, we would like to acknowledge the support of our beloved "outer" families in our efforts to explain the inner ones.

WHO IS THIS SPEAKING, PLEASE?

RECOGNIZING THE MEMBERS
OF YOUR INNER FAMILY

Multiplicity of mind is based on the idea that we all have various entities of the psyche, otherwise known as voices, subpersonalities, aspects, and so on, that express our most basic needs. For this book, we have identified nine common ones, ranging from the Body Regulator (the one that advocates for the basic biological needs of safety, stability, and balance) to the Meaning Maker (the one that sees the big picture and seeks purpose, harmony, and wholeness in life).

Each of these voices is going to sound different in each individual. However, they ask common questions and often have predictable responses in the ongoing internal monologue that each individual experiences. So how do you know which voice is talking? What are the likely expressions each voice would use in a given situation?

In this section we've listed utterances that are typical for each voice and some of the traits exhibited by those individuals for whom a particular voice speaks loudly.

AUTONOMY

- "I know what's best for me."
- "I'm my own person."
- "Don't compare me to her (or him)!"
- "I march to the beat of my own drummer."
- "People accept me for who I am."
- "If I don't look after myself, no one else will."
- "I am the author of my own life."
- "I won't live my life pleasing others."

Characteristics of one who has a strong voice of Autonomy:

- Is authentic.
- Is self-reliant.
- Is a self-starter.
- Enjoys being alone and enjoys working alone.

THE BODY REGULATOR

- "I need to take good care of myself."
- "No, I'm not staying up to watch *The Tonight Show*. It's important that I get enough sleep."
- "I think I should start work a half hour early so I have extra time to get in a power walk at lunch."

- "Get up! We've been in front of this computer for hours. I've read that all that sitting isn't good for your health."
- "Where's the nearest Whole Foods?"
- "Hang gliding? Bungee jumping? Are you kidding me? I don't take those kinds of risks. We could really get hurt."
- "Quit my job with the pension to start my own business? No way!"
- "I invest in my safety and security . . . not in some speculative stock."

Characteristics of one who has a strong Body Regulator:

- Invests in health daily.
- Eats healthy food most of the time.
- Enjoys exercise.
- Is prudent with finances.
- Rests and recharges frequently.
- Plays it safe.

CONFIDENCE

- "I think I can take on any challenge that comes my way."
- "I'm doing what I do well."
- "I'm pretty confident that I can . . ." (Complete the sentence.)

- "The new software system they just installed in my company? Yeah, I'm going to take the tutorial so that I can master that."
- "I know what my strengths are, and most of what I try to do plays to those strengths."
- "I think I can use my skills to help others."
- "As I look back over my life, I can see how my competence and my confidence have grown."

Characteristics of one who has a strong voice of Confidence:

- Has an upright body posture, a proud stance and demeanor, and a strong voice.
- Enjoys practicing new activities to build competence.
- Seeks healthy competition.
- Seeks ways to use strengths and abilities well.

THE CREATIVE

- "There's a different way to look at this problem and come up with a solution. We just have to figure out what it is."
- "I like thinking outside the box."
- "You always have to make time for fun and spontaneity."
- "Oh yes, I'm a bit of a daydreamer. I like to let my mind wander."
- "I love creative projects in which I get completely absorbed and lose track of time."

Characteristics of one who has a strong Creative voice:

- Loves humor and fun.
- Wants spontaneity and wishes to indulge impulses.
- Enjoys the creative process in any life domain, not just in writing, singing, painting, or other artistic pursuits (having a strong Creative subpersonality is not necessarily synonymous with having artistic talent).
- Wants to come up with new ideas to address life challenges.
- Prefers nonlinear thinking and activities.

THE CURIOUS ADVENTURER

- "The world is a fascinating place. There's never a dull moment."
- "Let's take that trail. We've never walked that way before."
- "I wonder what it's like to . . . ?" (Complete the sentence.)
- "I am so done with this. I need to shake things up."
- "No more of the same old, same old. Let's try something different."
- "A triathlon? Sure, I'd be up for trying that. How do I start training?"
- "I enjoy at least a little risk, uncertainty, and change, even if it means a little adversity."
- "A new restaurant? I'm in! Let's try it."

Characteristics of one who has a strong Curious Adventurer:

- ♦ Wants novel things, experiences, and projects.
- ♦ Is open to new ideas and experiences.
- ♦ Enjoys being curious.
- ♦ Gets excited about new opportunities and possibilities.

THE EXECUTIVE MANAGER

- ♦ "I spend time daily planning and completing my to-do lists."
- ♦ "I make sure I get my high-priority activities done each day."
- ♦ "I keep the main domains of my life organized."
- ♦ "I seek clarity in my thinking."
- ♦ "I move easily from nitty-gritty details to strategic thinking."
- ♦ "I am objective in my perspectives on myself, others, and the world."
- ♦ "I am a good self-regulator. I rein in my impulses and distractions to stay focused on key activities."

Characteristics of one who has a strong Executive Manager:

- ♦ Loves order and clarity.
- ♦ Finds order in chaos.
- ♦ Keeps well organized.
- ♦ Plans and prepares carefully.

THE RELATIONAL

- "I care a lot about the needs of others and helping them to get their needs met, sometimes before my needs are met."
- "I am empathetic when others are suffering."
- "I am self-compassionate when I am experiencing negative emotions."
- "I am loyal to my family, friends, and close colleagues."
- "I need loving relationships and invest in keeping them healthy."
- "I enjoy the company of others and learning about their lives."

Characteristics of one who has a strong Relational voice:

- Is empathetic and caring toward family, friends, and other close associates.
- Is a caregiver.
- Donates generously to help other people.
- Is trusting and loyal.

THE STANDARD SETTER

- "I want to achieve great things in my life."
- "I set a high bar for myself and others."
- "I want to be respected and treated fairly."
- "I want recognition for my achievements."
- "I want to impress other people."

Characteristics of one who has a strong Standard Setter:

- Is a high achiever.
- Pushes him- or herself hard and persists to complete difficult tasks.
- Is at least somewhat concerned with appearances, fame, and status.

THE MEANING MAKER

- "Why I am here?"
- "I stop to consider my greater purpose in life most days."
- "I often wonder what happens to us after we die."
- "Sometimes I wonder what it's all about."
- "I am grateful for what I have."
- "I am awed by life."

Characteristics of one who has a strong Meaning Maker:

- Looks beyond the immediate issue to see the bigger picture.
- Seeks wisdom and a wise perspective on life.
- Wants a higher purpose and to leave a legacy.
- Experiences gratitude for life's gifts.
- Identifies learning in adversity and tracks personal growth.

REFERENCES AND RESOURCES

THE MULTIPLICITY OF MIND HYPOTHESIS

The assertion of the existence of subpersonalities—a concept we also refer to as multiplicity of mind—began early in the twentieth century with Freud's description of the id, the ego, and the superego. John Rowan's book *Subpersonalities: The People Inside Us* explores the long history and diverse theories that support the existence of subpersonalities, thought to be enduring psychological structures that evolve over time. Subpersonalities integrate thoughts, emotions, needs, physiology, and behaviors. Rowan's working definition of a *subpersonality* is "a semi-permanent and semi-autonomous region of the personality capable of acting as a person."

Among the most active bodies of investigation and application of the concept of multiplicity of mind is the work of psychologist Richard Schwartz in developing the model of Internal Family Systems therapy. Applying radical empiricism, as he puts it, Schwartz has devoted more than twenty-five years to exploring inner dialogues among "parts" of the psyche. Schwartz, and thousands of therapists trained in Internal Family Systems therapy, help people invite their parts that are experiencing negative emotions to a mindful, meditation-like sit-down. The therapy session follows a winding trail to uncover small or large traumas and then unpacks the parts' interesting and often surprising narratives. From the vantage point of a Mindful Self, the client sits compassionately while experiencing the suffering of the parts and experiences a process designed to heal and release the burdens of the parts, which manifest as managers (self-protection role) and exiles (parts cut off from explicit memory as a result of a small or large trauma).

Thus far, models of subpersonalities have not proposed the existence of shared, universal subpersonalities. The clinical application of existing models allows clients to discover and engage their internal voices experientially and organically. The hypothesis supporting this book goes further, proposing that the psyche may have universal capacities, or subpersonalities, integrated and led by a central self. The strengths-based approach of such a universal structure offers a simpler tool for non-therapists to access and learn from their distinct inner voices as widely recognized universal capacities.

This book builds upon a hypothesis, advanced by our coauthor Margaret Moore, describing a strengths-based multiplicity of mind model:

1. We share a set of primary capacities, which may also be described as needs, drives, values, strengths, or capacities, generated by evolution, and which may manifest as subpersonalities; and
2. Each of these capacities has been validated as important to human well-being by a body of research or is being studied by scientists.

References and Resources: Thriving

Keyes, C. "The Mental Health Continuum: From Languishing to Flourishing in Life." *Journal of Health and Social Research* 43 (2002): 207–22.

Moore, M. "From Surviving to Thriving." *International Coaching Federation Coaching World* (blog), August 2014.

References and Resources: Multiplicity of Mind

Assagioli, R. *Psychosynthesis*. New York: Viking, 2006.

Mayer, J. "A Framework for the Classification of Personality Components." *Journal of Personality* 63, no. 4 (1995): 819–78.

Moore, M. "Coaching the Multiplicity of Mind: A Strengths-Based Model." *Global Advances in Health and Medicine* 2, no. 4 (2013): 78–84. doi: 10.7453/gahmj.13.030.

Rowan, J. *Subpersonalities: The People Inside Us*. London: Routledge, 1990.

Schwartz, R. *Internal Family Systems Therapy*. New York: Guilford Press, 1997. (For more on Internal Family Systems therapy, see www.selfleadership.org.)

Schwartz, R. "Message from Dick," in *Inside Out*, a blog by the Center for Self-Leadership, 2015.

Shadick, N. A., N. F. Sowell, M. L. Frits, S. M. Hoffman, S. A. Hartz, F. D. Booth, M. Sweezy et al. "A Randomized Controlled Trial of an Internal Family Systems–Based Psychotherapeutic Intervention on Outcomes in Rheumatoid Arthritis: A Proof-of-Concept Study." *Journal of Rheumatology* 40, no. 11 (2013): 1831–41. doi: 10.3899/jrheum.121465.

CHAPTER 1: THE NINE MEMBERS OF YOUR INNER FAMILY—AND ONE MINDFUL SELF

References and Resources: Mindfulness

Ives-Deliperi, V. "The Neural Substrates of Mindfulness: An fMRI Investigation." *Social Neuroscience* 6, no. 3 (2011): 231–42.

Vago, D. R., and D. A. Silbersweig. "Self-Awareness, Self-Regulation, and Self-Transcendence (S-ART): A Framework for Understanding the Neurobiological Mechanisms of Mindfulness." *Frontiers in Human Neuroscience* 6, article 296 (2012).

References and Resources: Self-Talk

Hendricksen, E. "Talking to Myself—Is That Normal?" *Scientific American,* August 6, 2014. http://www.scientificamerican.com /article/talking-to-myself-mdash-is-that-normal/.

Jabr, F. "Speak for Yourself." *Scientific American Mind,* January/February 2014.

Kross, E., and I. Grossmann. "Boosting Wisdom: Distance from the Self Enhances Wise Reasoning, Attitudes, and Behavior." *Journal of Experimental Psychology* 141, no. 1 (2012): 43–48.

Weintraub, P. "The Voice of Reason." *Psychology Today,* May 2015. https://www.psychologytoday.com/articles/201505/the-voice -reason?collection=1073568

References and Resources: Primary Capacities

Moore, M. "Coaching the Multiplicity of Mind: A Strengths-Based Model." *Global Advances in Health and Medicine* 2, no. 4 (2013): 78–84. doi: 10.7453/gahmj.13.030.

Moore, M. "From Surviving to Thriving." *International Coaching Federation Coaching World* (blog), August 2014.

CHAPTER 2: ROLL CALL! WHO'S WHO IN YOUR INNER FAMILY

Discussion

The description of the evolutionary origins of the nine capacities was developed by coauthor Margaret Moore to demonstrate how these capacities may have emerged from the evolutionary path of living organisms over billions of years on planet Earth.

References and Resources

Moore, M. "Coaching the Multiplicity of Mind: A Strengths-Based Model." *Global Advances in Health and Medicine* 2, no. 4 (2013): 78–84. doi: 10.7453/gahmj.13.030.

Moore, M. "From Surviving to Thriving." *International Coaching Federation Coaching World* (blog), August 2014.

Roth, V. *Divergent.* New York: HarperCollins, 2014.

CHAPTER 3: MEET YOUR EMOTIONS

Discussion

Katherine Peil characterizes emotions as perhaps the first sensory system to have emerged in human beings and asserts that they served the function of self-regulation. Emotions then provide self-relevant sensory information concerning optimally adaptive states for the organism in its immediate environment. Negative emotions can hence be decoded as signals that needs are being unmet, such as needs for relatedness or confidence, and positive emotions serve as signals that needs are being met, such as needs for novelty or creative expression.

References and Resources

Fredrickson, B. "Updated Thinking on Positivity Ratios." *American Psychologist* 68, no. 9 (2013): 814–22. doi: 10.1037/a0033584.

Hayes, S., K. Strosahl, and K. Wilson. *Acceptance and Commitment Therapy: The Process and Practice of Mindful Change.* 2nd ed. New York: Guilford Press, 2011.

Kashdan, T., and M. Steger. "Curiosity and Pathways to Well-Being and Meaning in Life: Traits, States, and Everyday Behaviors." *Motivation and Emotion* 31, no. 3 (2007): 159–73.

Lieberman, M. D., N. I. Eisenberger, M. J. Crockett, S. M. Tom, J. H. Pfeifer, and B. M. Way. "Putting Feelings into Words: Affect Labeling Disrupts Amygdala Activity in Response to Affective Stimuli." *Psychological Science* 18, no. 5 (2007): 421–28.

Macknik, S., and S. Martinez-Conde. "Is Pain a Construct of the Mind?" *Scientific American,* September 2013. http://www.scientificamerican.com/article/is-pain-construct-of-mind/.

Neff, K. D., and K. A. Dahm. "Self-Compassion: What It Is, What It Does, and How It Relates to Mindfulness." In *Handbook of Mindfulness and Self-Regulation,* edited by B. Ostafin, M. Robinson, and B. Meier, 121–37. New York: Springer, 2015.

Peil, K. T. "Emotion: The Self-Regulatory Sense." *Global Advances in Health & Medicine* 3, no. 2 (2014): 80–108.

CHAPTER 4: AUTONOMY

Discussion

Self-determination theory (SDT) also addresses primary human needs and well-being. SDT was developed by Edward Deci and Richard Ryan at the University of Rochester over the past thirty years, and it is the most-studied theory of human motivation, having been explored in more than one thousand published papers to date. The theory posits the existence of three basic psychological needs that together are universally essential (consistent across cultures) for ongoing psychological growth, integrity, and well-being. Those three basic needs are autonomy, competence, and relatedness.

Deci and Ryan note: "The starting point for SDT is the postulate that humans are active, growth-oriented organisms who are naturally inclined toward integration of their psychic elements into a unified sense of self and integration of themselves into larger social structures. SDT suggests that it is part of the adaptive design of the human organism to engage [in] interesting activities, to exercise capacities, to pursue connectedness in social groups, and to integrate intrapsychic and interpersonal experiences into a relative unity."

Deci and Ryan describe autonomy, that is, the need to be autonomous and to have meaningful choice, rather than to be controlled, as the primary organismic drive. In the face of external control, this drive can lead to resistance or defiance, as a means to assert self-interest and thus avoid this external control. Deci and Ryan's self-determination theory "argues that developing a sense of autonomy (and competence) is critical to the processes of internalization and integration, through which a person comes to self-regulate and sustain behaviors conducive to health and well-being."

References and Resources

Chen, B., M. Vansteenkiste, W. Beyers, L. Boone, E. L. Deci, J. Van der Kaap-Deeder, B. Duriez et al. "Basic Psychological Need Satisfaction, Need Frustration, and Need Strength across Four Cultures." *Motivation and Emotion* 39, no. 2 (2015): 216–36. doi 10.1007/s11031-014-9450-1.

Deci, E. L. *Why We Do What We Do: Understanding Self-Motivation.* New York: Penguin, 1995.

Deci, E. L., and R. M. Ryan. *Handbook of Self-Determination Research.* New York: University of Rochester Press, 2004.

Deci, E. L., and R. M. Ryan. "The 'What' and the 'Why' of Goal Pursuits: Human Needs and the Self-Determination of Behavior." *Psychological Inquiry* 11 (2000): 227–68.

Ryan R. M., H. Patrick, E. L. Deci, and G. C. Williams. "Facilitating Health Behaviour Change and Its Maintenance: Interventions based on Self-Determination Theory." *The European Health Psychologist* 10 (March 2008).

Video (toddler). https://www.youtube.com/v/G8FU18NkVK4.

CHAPTER 5: THE BODY REGULATOR

Discussion

Maslow's hierarchy of needs is a psychological theory proposed by Abraham Maslow that at its base includes physiological needs, that is, the physical requirements for human survival; and safety and security needs, including physical, health, and financial safety and security.

Along with all living organisms, humans have a primary need for a healthy and calm equilibrium of their physiological systems—a need to move from chaos to homeostasis over and over. As Stephen W. Porges illustrates in his polyvagal theory, our bodies seek a balance of exertion and rest (recharging). They strive for homeostasis, stability, and a healthy autonomic nervous system, balancing sympathetic (stress) and parasympathetic (rest and recover) activity. By listening to the body's signals, engaging in what one might call "body intelligence," we can discern when it's time to calm the nervous system, which calms the mind and improves brain function in the short term, and delays disease and early death in the long term.

References and Resources

Gavin, J., and M. Moore. "Body Intelligence: A Guide to Self-Attunement." *IDEA Fitness Journal* 7, no. 11 (2010). http://www.ideafit.com/fitness-library/body-intelligence-a-guide-to.

Maslow, A. *Motivation and Personality*. New York: Harper & Row, 1954.

Porges, S. W. "The Polyvagal Perspective." *Biological Psychology* 74, no. 2 (2007): 116–43.

CHAPTER 6: CONFIDENCE AND THE STANDARD SETTER

Discussion: Confidence

The extensive literature describing self-efficacy as a primary psychological construct, including Deci and Ryan's determination of competence as one of the three primary organismic drives (along with autonomy and relatedness), suggests that one's belief in one's abilities and one's desire to be strong, confident, competent, and effective is a primary capacity. One's sense of strength, or empowerment, is a key determinant of behavior and effectiveness. It varies widely and is domain specific to myriad life activities and social environments. According to Bandura's social cognitive theory, "the beliefs one holds regarding one's power to affect situations strongly influences both the power one has to face challenges competently and the choices a person is most likely to make. These effects are particularly apparent, and compelling, with regard to behaviors affecting health."

References and Resources: Confidence

Bandura, A. *Self-Efficacy: The Exercise of Control.* New York: Freeman, 1997.

Chen, B., M. Vansteenkiste, W. Beyers, L. Boone, E. L. Deci, J. Van der Kaap-Deeder, B. Duriez et al. "Basic Psychological Need Satisfaction, Need Frustration, and Need Strength across Four Cultures." *Motivation and Emotion* 39, no. 2 (2015) 216–36. doi 10.1007/s11031-014-9450-1.

Luszczynska, A., and R. Schwarzer. "Social Cognitive Theory." In *Predicting Health Behaviour,* edited by M. Conner and P. Norman, 127–69. 2nd ed. Buckingham, UK: Open University Press, 2005.

Ryan, R. M. "Psychological Needs and the Facilitation of Integrative Processes." *Journal of Personality* 63, no. 3 (1995): 397–427.

Stajkovic, A., and F. Luthans. "Self-Efficacy and Work-Related Performance: A Meta-Analysis." *Psychological Bulletin* 124, no. 2 (1998): 240–61.

Tomkins, S. "Interest-Excitement." In *Affect Imagery Consciousness: The Complete Edition: Two Volumes,* 188. New York: Springer, 2008.

Video. *The Way to Happiness Video: Be Competent.* https://www.youtube.com/v/L-1nhV6MaJ8.

White, R. W. "Motivation Reconsidered: The Concept of Competence." *Psychological Review* 66, no. 5 (1959): 297–333.

Discussion: The Standard Setter

The National Association for Self-Esteem (NASE) combines both competence and worthiness in its definition of *self-esteem.* This book and model tease apart these two aspects of the psyche. If we do that with this definition, then the NASE characterizes self-esteem as "being worthy of happiness." The worthiness is tied to whether or not a person lives up to certain fundamental human values, such as finding meanings that foster human growth and making commitments to them in a way that leads to a sense of integrity and satisfaction. Other elements include tolerance and respect for others, acceptance of responsibility for one's actions, integrity, and pride in one's accomplishments. People have healthy or authentic self-esteem because they trust their own being to be life affirming, constructive, responsible, and trustworthy.

The term *self-esteem* includes cognitive, affective, and behavioral elements. It is cognitive as one consciously thinks about oneself as one considers the discrepancy between one's ideal self, the person one wishes to be, and the perceived self or the realistic appraisal of how one sees oneself. The affective element refers to the feelings or emotions that one has when considering that discrepancy. The behavioral aspects of self-esteem are manifested in such behaviors as assertiveness, goal pursuit, resilience, decisiveness, and respectfulness toward others.

As the most social animals on the planet, humans share a primary need for respect, approval, appreciation, validation, and fair treatment. We want to be accepted and valued by our tribes. This capacity allows us to set the bar or standard, to set goals for our performance, and then to evaluate and judge our performance, and that of others, across all domains of life, from getting good grades at school to dying well. "Am I good enough?" it asks. At its worst, this capacity is difficult to please. It can be an inner critic, scanning for flaws and faults, or a perfectionist, ever raising the bar.

References and Resources: The Standard Setter

Baumeister, R., J. Campbell, J. Krueger, and K. Vohs. "Does High Self-Esteem Cause Better Performance, Interpersonal

Success, Happiness, or Healthier Lifestyles?" *Psychological Science in the Public Interest* 4, no. 1 (2003): 1–44.

National Association for Self-Esteem. http://www.self-esteem -nase.org.

Rosenberg's Self-Esteem Scale. http://www.wwnorton.com/college /psych/psychsci/media/rosenberg.htm.

CHAPTER 7: THE CURIOUS ADVENTURER

Discussion

In his body of work on neural mechanisms of emotion, Jaak Panksepp, an affective neuroscientist, explores the "seeking system" in animals and humans and summarizes its features:

- ◆ Urges us to find resources and avoid dangers and threats.
- ◆ Energizes all our capabilities, from basic impulses to intellectualizing.
- ◆ Feeds the appetite for novelty and learning.
- ◆ Makes the mundane exciting.

Silvan Tomkins, a theorist on emotion and emotional expression, notes in the 2008 book *Affect Imagery Consciousness: The Complete Edition:* "The interrelationships between the affect of interest and the functions of thought and memory are so extensive that absence of the affective support of interest would jeopardize intellectual development no less than destruction of brain tissue."

In his 2012 article "Reconsidering the Neuroevolutionary Framework of the SEEKING System," psychologist Todd Kashdan asserts that curiosity is a primary driver of human well-being, writing, "From an evolutionary perspective, the acquisition of new experiences and knowledge is essential for survival." Kashdan distinguishes between bottom-up curiosity, resulting from a novel or unexpected event, and triggering a sense of wonder and a desire for exploration; and top-down curiosity, purposely possessing a state of awareness and openness in any given moment.

References and Resources

Kashdan, T. *Curious?: Discover the Missing Ingredient to a Fulfilling Life*. New York: HarperCollins, 2009.

Kashdan, T. "The Power of Curiosity." *Experience Life* (2010). Retrieved from https://experiencelife.com/article/the-power-of-curiosity/.

Kashdan, T. "Reconsidering the Neuroevolutionary Framework of the SEEKING System: Emphasizing Context instead of Positivity." *Neuropsychoanalysis* 14, no. 1 (2012): 46–50.

Panksepp, J. *Affective Neuroscience: The Foundations of Human and Animal Emotions*. New York: Oxford University Press, 2004.

Tomkins, S. *Exploring Affect: The Selected Writings of Silvan S. Tomkins*. Edited by E. Virginia Demos. Cambridge: Cambridge University Press, 1995.

Tomkins, S. "Interest-Excitement." In *Affect Imagery Consciousness: The Complete Edition: Two Volumes*, 188. New York: Springer, 2008.

CHAPTER 8: THE CREATIVE AND THE EXECUTIVE MANAGER

Discussion: The Creative

Creativity is often described as the ability to think outside the box and invent or design new ideas and technologies. Creative processes are generative, imaginative, and spontaneous, deploying nonlinear thinking processes. Creative processes are at work in brainstorming, playing games, and being impulsive. Creative flow states, which Mihaly Csikszentmihalyi (pronounced cheek-sent-me-hi) describes as key to optimal well-being, are those moments when we are engrossed in an activity and are enjoying it so much that we lose track of time. Without undue effort—in fact when there is a mild defocusing of attentional resources—we execute the activity to the best of our abilities.

In her book *Your Creative Brain*, Harvard psychologist Shelley Carson notes that the brain activation pattern for defocused idea-generating activity shows significant activation of the right prefrontal cortex, although the creative processes progress through multiple stages and engage many brain regions.

Creativity is a major topic across a wide spectrum of scientific endeavor. In their chapter on creativity in *Character Strengths and Virtues: A Handbook and Classification*, Christopher Peterson and Martin Seligman assert that "[i]t is difficult to conceive a single major theoretical orientation that has not tried to make a contribution to our understanding of creativity."

References and Resources: The Creative

Carson, S. *Your Creative Brain: Seven Steps to Maximize Imagination, Productivity, and Innovation in Your Life.* San Francisco: Jossey-Bass, 2010.

Csikszentmihalyi, M. *Flow: The Psychology of Optimal Experience.* New York: Harper Perennial, 2008.

Peterson, C., and M. Seligman. *Character Strengths and Virtues: A Handbook and Classification.* New York: Oxford University Press, 2004.

Discussion: The Executive Manager

Executive functions is an umbrella term for the regulation and control of a complex set of cognitive processes, residing partly in the left prefrontal cortex, while drawing on other brain regions. These processes regulate a person's ability to organize thoughts and activities, manage emotions, prioritize tasks, manage time efficiently, and make decisions. They are involved in solving problems; analyzing information; being productive; getting things done efficiently; creating plans, goals, and to-do lists, and marshaling resources to accomplish tasks. They direct focus and attention on the task at hand and regulate emotions, impulses, and distractions.

References and Resources: The Executive Manager

Elliott, R. "Executive Functions and Their Disorders: Imaging in Clinical Neuroscience." *British Medical Bulletin* 65, no. 1 (2003): 49–59.

Hammerness, P., M. Moore, and J. Hanc. *Organize Your Mind, Organize Your Life*. New York: Harlequin, 2012.

CHAPTER 9: THE RELATIONAL

Discussion

As noted in the section on autonomy, self-determination research has identified relatedness as one of three innate psychological needs vital to well-being. Feeling connected, serving others, taking care of others, loving and being loved, belonging, and being compassionate and kind are important sources of human well-being.

In *Love 2.0: How Our Supreme Emotion Affects Everything We Feel, Think, Do, and Become*, Barbara Fredrickson encourages us to "make love all day long," that is, to infuse each moment in another's company with our full attention, our head and heart in it together. In addition to simply making us feel good, sharing positive emotions with others creates micromoments of connection, which calm the nervous system and improve brain function. Over time, these micromoments accumulate and help delay both disease and early death.

References and Resources

Chen, B., M. Vansteenkiste, W. Beyers, L. Boone, E. L. Deci, J. Van der Kaap-Deeder, B. Duriez et al. "Basic Psychological Need Satisfaction, Need Frustration, and Need Strength across Four Cultures." *Motivation and Emotion* 39, no. 2 (2015): 216–36. doi 10.1007/s11031-014-9450-1.

Fredrickson, B. *Love 2.0: How Our Supreme Emotion Affects Everything We Feel, Think, Do, and Become.* New York: Hudson Street Press, 2013.

Ryan, R. M. "Psychological Needs and the Facilitation of Integrative Processes." *Journal of Personality* 63, no. 3 (1995): 397–427.

CHAPTER 10: THE MEANING MAKER

Discussion

Clinical psychologist Paul Wong is the most passionate spokesperson for the importance of making meaning and purpose beyond oneself in each moment, in each domain of life, and over the arc of a lifetime. In his chapter "Viktor Frankl's Meaning-Seeking Model and Positive Psychology" in *Meaning in Positive and Existential Psychology,* Wong keeps alive the legendary psychiatrist and Holocaust survivor's story, told in *Man's Search for*

Meaning, of how having an unshakable purpose was essential to surviving four concentration camps.

After the Holocaust experience, Frankl developed "logotherapy" to help people find meaning through doing good deeds, experiencing values, and experiencing suffering. Logotherapy involves creating meaning in one's life after the experience of loss and tragedy. Frankl, who lost everything and everyone he loved during the Holocaust, was able to create meaning out of his situation by valuing life. This therapy helps people make meaning out of their losses, as well as reestablish the meaning of their own life in order to cope with mortality and loss.

A sense of a higher meaning or purpose is a potent source of life fuel, especially when times are tough. For example, a team of researchers at Rush Alzheimer's Disease Center and Rush University Medical Center in Chicago found that a sense of life purpose significantly improves cognitive function in people with Alzheimer's disease.

References and Resources

Boyle, P. A., A. S. Buchman, R. S. Wilson, L. Yu, J. A. Schneider, and D. A. Bennett. "Effect of Purpose in Life on the Relation between Alzheimer Disease Pathologic Changes on Cognitive Function in Advanced Age." *Archives of General Psychiatry* 69, no. 5 (2012): 499–505.

Wong. P. *International Journal of Existential Psychology & Psychotherapy* 5, no. 1 (2014).

Wong, P. "Viktor Frankl's Meaning-Seeking Model and Positive Psychology." In *Meaning in Positive and Existential Psychology,* edited by A. Batthyany and P. Russo-Netzer, 149–84. New York: Springer, 2014.

INDEX

ABOUT THE AUTHORS

MARGARET MOORE, MBA, aka Coach Meg, is the founder and CEO of Wellcoaches Corporation which, in strategic partnership with the American College of Sports Medicine, has trained more than ten thousand health and wellness coaches in forty-five countries. She is coauthor of the first coaching textbook in healthcare, the *Coaching Psychology Manual,* and coauthor of the 2012 bestseller *Organize Your Mind, Organize Your Life,* and a companion course at www.organizeyourmind.com.

Margaret is cofounder and codirector of the Institute of Coaching at McLean Hospital, a Harvard Medical School affiliate, and codirector of the annual Coaching in Leadership & Healthcare conference offered by Harvard Medical School. Margaret teaches a coaching psychology program at Harvard University Extension School. She cofounded and coleads the National Consortium for Credentialing Health & Wellness Coaches, delivering national standards and certification for health and wellness coaches. Margaret, whose executive coaching practice is now dedicated mainly to healthcare leaders, has helped thousands of individuals transform their lives and well-being.

EDWARD PHILLIPS, MD, is Assistant Professor of Physical Medicine and Rehabilitation at Harvard Medical School and is founder and director of the Institute of Lifestyle Medicine (ILM) at Spaulding Rehabilitation Hospital (www.Instituteof LifestyleMedicine.org).

In 2015 Phillips began his role as Chief of Physical Medicine & Rehabilitation Service at the VA Boston Healthcare System. Additionally, Phillips is a Fellow of the American College of Sports Medicine and serves on the executive council that developed and leads the Exercise is Medicine global initiative. He is coauthor of *ACSM's Exercise is Medicine: A Clinician's Guide to Exercise Prescription.*

Phillips is an active clinician and researcher who speaks and consults nationally, guiding a broad-based effort to reduce lifestyle-related death, disease, and costs through clinician-directed interventions with patients. The President's Council on Fitness, Sports and Nutrition has recognized both Dr. Phillips and the ILM with its Community Leadership Award.

JOHN HANC has written or coauthored fourteen books, including *Organize Your Mind, Organize Your Life;* the award-winning 2015 book *The Ultra Mindset,* written with ultra-distance endurance champion Travis Macy; and his own award-winning memoir on running the Antarctica Marathon, *The Coolest Race on Earth.* A longtime health and fitness writer, Hanc is a frequent contributor to the *New York Times,* a contributing editor for *Runner's World* magazine, and a contributing writer for *Smithsonian.* He is an associate professor at the New York Institute of Technology in Old Westbury, New York, where he teaches journalism and writing, and is a faculty member at Harvard Medical School's annual writing conference for healthcare professionals, Achieving Healthcare Leadership and Outcomes through Writing and Publishing.

ALSO AVAILABLE

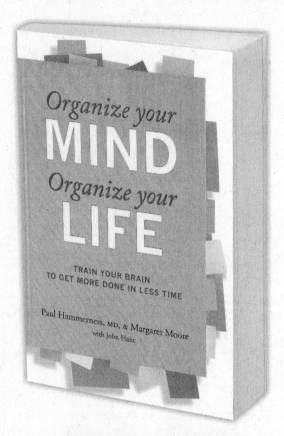

ORGANIZE YOUR MIND, ORGANIZE YOUR LIFE
Train Your Brain to Get More Done in Less Time
Available in Paperback and Ebook

The key to a less hectic, less stressful life is not in simply organizing your desk, but in organizing your mind. Dr. Paul Hammerness, a Harvard Medical School psychiatrist, describes the latest neuroscience research on the brain's extraordinary built-in system of organization. Margaret Moore, an executive wellness coach and codirector of the Institute of Coaching, translates the science into solutions.